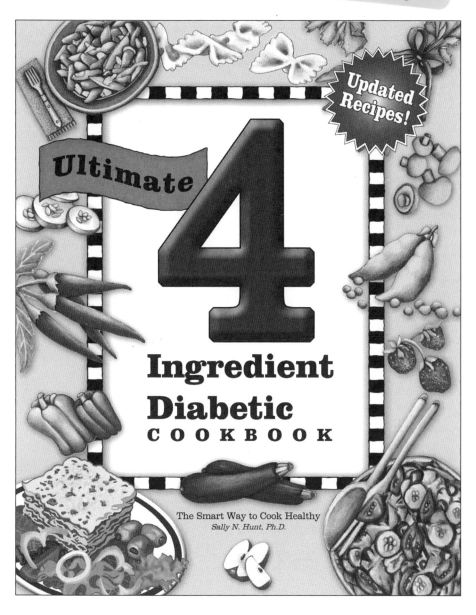

Ultimate

4

Ingredient
Diabetic
COOKBOOK

Updated Recipes!

The Smart Way to Cook Healthy
Sally N. Hunt, Ph.D.

Cookbook Resources, LLC
Highland Village, Texas

Ultimate 4 Ingredient Diabetic Cookbook
The Smart Way to Cook Healthy

Printed November 2012

International Standard Book Number: ISBN 978-1-59769-204-5

Library of Congress Control Number: 2011932624

Library of Congress Cataloging-in-Publication Data

    Hunt, Sally N.
      Ultimate 4 ingredient diabetic cookbook : the smart way to cook healthy / Sally N. Hunt.
        p. cm.
      Includes bibliographical references and index.
      ISBN 978-1-59769-000-3
      1. Diabetes--Diet therapy--Recipes. 2. Quick and easy cooking. I. Title. II. Title: Ultimate four ingredient diabetic cookbook.

    RC662.H868 2010
    641.5'6314--dc22

                        2010022621

Cover and Illustrations by Nancy Bohanan and Nancy Griffith

Edited, Designed and Published in the United States of America
and Manufactured in China by
Cookbook Resources, LLC
541 Doubletree Drive
Highland Village, Texas 75077

Toll free 866-229-2665

www.cookbookresources.com

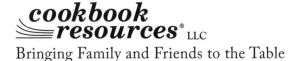

Bringing Family and Friends to the Table

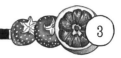
About the Cookbook

U*ltimate 4 Ingredient Diabetic Cookbook* is a cookbook of 4-ingredient recipes. What could be simpler? With fewer ingredients in the recipes, you will spend less time shopping and less time in the kitchen.

This cookbook is not just for individuals with diabetes, but for anyone seeking a healthier way of eating. You will not need to buy expensive "diabetic" food products, because locally available fresh, frozen and canned foods that you enjoy are included in the recipes. Emphasis is on fresh fruits, vegetables, whole grains, lean meats, and low-fat milk products.

Each recipe has a "Nutrition Facts" label – listing calories and amounts of fat, cholesterol, sodium, total carbohydrate, dietary fiber, sugars and protein. The label format is similar to the one found on food products, which you may already be using effectively. If you are not familiar with the nutrition label, this cookbook will help you understand how to use those facts. You will be able to monitor your carbohydrate and sugar intake and practice "carb counting" to improve overall health.

Recipes and ingredients have been carefully analyzed using the most current nutritional information and the U.S.D.A. National Nutrient Database. Food products were chosen to reduce calories, fat, cholesterol and levels of sodium. The ingredients were carefully selected to keep total carbohydrates and sugars low, while ensuring adequate amounts of dietary fiber and protein.

This cookbook is not intended as a substitute for the advice of your health professional. Always consult your doctor or nutritionist for specific instructions for diabetic meal plans or weight loss programs.

Preparing and eating nutritious foods is only one aspect contributing to your overall health needs. The recipes provide a simple, easy way to keep unhealthy ingredients low and focus on all the good-for-you foods. It's important to follow the dietary guidelines set by your health professionals. But, remember, YOU are the key in managing a healthy food plan and lifestyle.

Wishing you good health and well being!

Sally N. Hunt, Ph.D.

About the Author

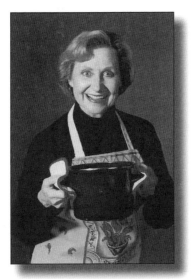

Sally N. Hunt, Ph.D.

Sally N. Hunt earned her Ph.D. at Texas Woman's University, M.S. at Northwestern State University of Louisiana, and B.S. at the University of Oklahoma. Her areas of study and research were in Home Economics Secondary Education, with concentration in foods and nutrition.

For 25 years, she was a Teacher Educator and Administrator at the university level. Hunt taught home economics, secondary education and foods and nutrition classes from high school through college levels. She has appeared on local television programs and the QVC network.

Her published cookbooks include *Easy Diabetic Recipes, 365 Vegetarian Recipes, Easy Diabetic Cooking with 4 Ingredients,* and *Easy Healthy Cooking with 4 Ingredients.*

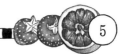

Dedication

Cookbook Resources' mission is

Bringing Family and Friends to the Table.

We recognize the importance of shared meals as a means of building family bonds with memories and traditions that will last a lifetime. At mealtimes we share more than food. We share ourselves.

This cookbook is dedicated with gratitude and respect to all those who show their love by making home-cooked meals and bringing family and friends to the table.

The Publisher

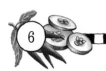

Contents

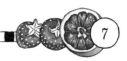
About Diabetes

More than 17 million Americans have diabetes. That's more than 6 percent of the U.S. population. Why is diabetes such a problem in the U.S.? Health experts agree that diabetes has spread, in large part, due to high-fat and high-calorie food intake and lack of exercise, which leads to obesity. Obesity is a major risk factor for diabetes.

Understanding Diabetes

First, it's important to understand glucose and insulin. Glucose, a form of sugar, is the main fuel the body needs for energy. Glucose is made when the food you eat breaks down during digestion. It travels through the bloodstream and enters the body's cells with the help of insulin.

Insulin is a hormone made in the pancreas and is essential to transferring glucose into cells. Diabetes develops when insulin is not available in adequate amounts. Without insulin, too much glucose stays in the blood and causes the complications of diabetes. About 90 percent of people with diabetes have type 2 diabetes that occurs when cells resist insulin, and glucose does not transfer easily into cells.

Some Helpful Tools

The "Diabetes Food Guide Pyramid" is a visual pyramid that divides food into six groups based on similar nutrition. As part of your personal food plan, your health professional may use the pyramid to help you learn about food groupings and will give you guidelines for specific number of servings from each group.

"Carbohydrate Counting" is a newer approach to meal planning for diabetics. People are encouraged to eat consistent amounts of carbohydrate at meals and snacks at similar times each day. It is a plan where people learn how to accurately count grams of carbohydrate from recipes and labels and keep track of daily intake. Refer to "What Do I Eat Now?" by Geil and Ross, available at www.diabetes.org.

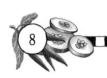

"Create Your Plate" is a simple and effective way to focus on portion sizes. Using your dinner plate, fill half your plate with non-starchy vegetables such as spinach, cabbage, green beans, and broccoli. Fill one-fourth of your plate with starchy foods such as rice, pasta, corn, potatoes, and whole grain foods. Fill the remaining one-fourth of your plate with meat and meat substitutes, such as chicken, lean meat and fish. An 8-ounce glass of fat-free milk is also recommended to add to your meal. Refer to www.diabetes.org.

The American Diabetic Association's "Exchange Lists" are foods grouped together because they are alike in amounts of carbohydrate, protein, fat and calories. You can exchange one food for another in the same group, such as exchanging a slice of bread for ½ cup cooked cereal. Refer to the publication,"Exchange Lists for Meal Planning," available at www.diabetes.org.

The U.S.D.A. has developed an online source tool called "My Pyramid," which is based on "Dietary Guidelines for Americans." The information is reader-friendly, continuously updated, and interactive for planning your personal health needs. Locate the program at www.mypyramid.gov.

Nutrition information on the internet may not originate from reliable sources. Ask yourself, who is responsible for the Web site? When was it last updated? Where is it coming from? Addresses ending in "gov", "edu", or "org" generally provide reliable information. Why is the site giving you information? Lastly, ask, is the message in line with other reliable sources?

Reliable Sources

American Diabetic Association.   www.diabetes.org

American Dietetic Association.   www.eatright.org

American Heart Association.   www.americanheart.org

Department of Agriculture (USDA).   www.usda.gov

Food and Drug Administration (FDA).   www.fda.gov

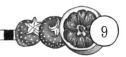

About Ingredients

Bread and Bread Products

Grains can be whole or refined; whole grains contain the entire grain kernel, as found in whole wheat bread or oatmeal. Many valuable nutrients are removed when grains are refined as in white flour. Whole grain and whole wheat products are recommended for the recipes t hat include breads such as English muffins, pita bread, flatbread and tortillas.

Broths

Select canned chicken broth that is 98% fat-free and reduced in sodium. Beef and vegetable broths also come fat-free and reduced-sodium. You can also find sodium-free chicken and beef broth seasonings and bouillon cubes. If you have the time, homemade broths, without additives, would be excellent.

Chicken and Turkey

Chicken is high in protein, low in fat and cholesterol and contains zero carbs, making it a winning choice for healthy eating. For many chicken recipes, "boneless, skinless chicken breast halves" are used. Convenient, packaged boneless, skinless chicken breasts are more expensive than the bone-in chicken breasts. You can save money by cutting and boning the chicken breasts at home. A sharp boning knife and a little patience will be worth the money saved.

Ground turkey breast, turkey cutlets and turkey sausage are also ingredients used. Check ground turkey labels to be sure you buy (white) ground turkey breast. Cooked turkey tends to be dry, so cook just until no longer pink.

Eggs and Egg Substitutes

Use large eggs when eggs are called for as an ingredient. Egg whites separated from fresh whole eggs are also used. Refrigerated cholesterol-free liquid egg substitutes and liquid egg whites are good substitutes for whole eggs. One-fourth cup liquid egg substitute is equal to one egg. Consult the manufacturer for uses of egg substitutes in cooking and baking.

The American Heart Association recommends that adults limit their cholesterol intake to no more than 300mg a day. Since one large egg contains 212mg of cholesterol, most of us need to limit our weekly intake of whole eggs.

Fruit

Many recipes include fresh fruit. Unfortunately, there isn't one rule for determining the ripeness of fruit – it varies from fruit to fruit. Some fruits such as grapes and pineapple don't ripen after they've been picked. Other fruit such as peaches and cantaloupe ripen in color, texture and juiciness after picking. A good rule is to buy fruits in season when they are most delicious; otherwise choose canned fruit that is canned in water or light syrup.

How much fruit can I eat each day? Diabetic food guidelines specify 2 to 4 servings – with serving sizes of 1 small to medium whole fruit, ½ cup of fresh or canned fruit or ¼ cup dried fruit. Each fruit serving has about 15 grams carbohydrate and 60 calories.

Meat

Choose lean cuts of beef for recipes for fajitas, chili, stew, roasts and steaks. Trim the meat and follow the low-fat cooking techniques. In particular, you need to pay attention to portion sizes of beef.

By reading the food labels on meat, you can determine the percentages of lean meat and fat as well as calories. The following

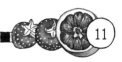

chart gives you specific information concerning the percentages in 3½ ounces (100g) of ground beef.

Percentages of Lean Meat and Fat (3.5 oz; 100g)	Calories
95% lean meat, 5% fat	137
90% lean meat, 10% fat	176
85% lean meat, 15% fat	215
80% lean meat, 20% fat	254

There are also recipes for lean cuts of pork – pork tenderloin, pork chops and roasts. Trim the fat before cooking and use the suggested cooking methods. You will find several slow cooker recipes for pork such as stews and pulled pork.

Milk and Cheese

Health guidelines for dairy products are for adults to consume 3 cups per day of fat-free or low-fat milk or milk products. Fat-free, reduced-fat and whole milk all contain 12g carbohydrate and 8g protein but differ in amounts of fat and calories. One cup fat-free milk has 0 to 3g fat and 100 calories compared to 8g fat and 160 calories in 1 cup whole milk. Fat-free yogurt, plain or flavored with an artificial sweetener, in 6-ounce portions, is equivalent to 1 cup fat-free milk.

Purchase fat-free or reduced-fat cream cheese, ricotta, cottage cheese and sour cream. Buy harder cheese like cheddar, Monterey Jack and Colby-Jack in block form and grate it yourself. Feta and blue cheeses come in crumbled form. Freshly grated parmesan cheese is much fresher-tasting than the dry, powdery form in shaker cans.

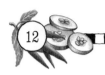

12

Ultimate 4 Ingredient Diabetic Cookbook

Nonstick Cooking Spray

Nonstick cooking spray is an essential ingredient for this cookbook. Grocery shelves have a variety of cooking sprays – olive oil, canola, butter, and regular nonstick sprays. Keep your preferred spray handy for the many recipes calling for "sprayed" skillets and "sprayed" baking dishes.

Oils

Choosing oils gets more complicated every day, due to so much information about *trans*-fats, saturated fats, mono- and polyunsaturated fats. Olive and canola oils in moderate amounts are used in recipes such as salad dressings and marinades. Experts consider the more expensive cold-pressed extra virgin olive oil the best choice, but you may prefer a lighter tasting olive oil. Frequently, nonstick cooking sprays replace oils to keep calories and fats in check. There are a few recipes that use small amounts of butter as an ingredient, mainly for flavor.

Peppers

What's the difference between green, yellow and red bell peppers? Green bell peppers are harvested before they are fully ripe, which is one reason they are less expensive. Orange and yellow peppers are ripened green peppers. Red peppers are more mature than the others and have a sweeter taste. Nutritionally, red peppers have 1½ times more vitamin C and 8 times more vitamin A than do green peppers.

You'll find several recipes using fresh jalapeño and poblano chilies. Most people are familiar with the flavorful, fairly hot jalapeño chile. When preparing jalapeño chilies, it is a good idea to use rubber gloves when cutting the pepper to avoid skin and eye irritations from the seeds. On the other hand, poblano is a mild, non-threatening pepper to prepare. Try the recipes using poblano chilies to experience a different chile flavor. See "Sausage Cheese-Stuffed Poblanos," p. 196, and "Poblano Chilies with Cheese," p. 134.

Fresh New Mexico or California (Anaheim) green chiles are excellent choices for cooking. Prior to use in recipes, roast the fresh chiles to remove the skins. Canned green chiles are a great convenience, both diced and whole, usually in 4-ounce cans.

Salt and Pepper

Table salt is NOT used in the recipes. Most of us reach for the salt shaker by habit, forgetting the sodium levels already in most of the foods we eat. Add salt sparingly, if at all, or use salt substitutes. Health experts recommend sodium levels between 1,200mg and 2,300 to 2,400mg per day, which is about one teaspoon of table salt. Pepper is also not specified in the recipes; however, use of pepper is your choice. Freshly ground peppercorns provide fresh, lively flavor in recipes.

Sugar Substitutes

Sugar substitutes are called non-nutritive sweeteners because they provide virtually no energy. Individuals use sugar substitutes to help them limit calories and minimize sugar intake.

In this cookbook, when you see "sugar substitute equal to 2 teaspoons sugar," it refers to the amount of sugar substitute that is equal to the SWEETNESS in 2 teaspoons sugar, not necessarily the same volume as 2 teaspoons of sugar.

Now on grocery shelves is a brown sugar-sugar substitute blend – half brown sugar and half sugar substitute. Since it is twice as sweet, use ½ cup for every cup of pure brown sugar. Since it is expensive, regular brown sugar in small amounts may be your best choice.

The FDA has approved safety of these low- or no-calorie sweeteners

Sugar Substitute	Some Brand Names	Details
Saccharin	Sweet'N Low® Sugar Twin®	Saccharin can be used to sweeten both hot and cold foods.
Aspartame	NutraSweet® Equal®	High temperatures can decrease sweetness of aspartame. Contact the manufacturer for recommended use of aspartame in baking and cooking.
Acesulfame K (potassium)	Sweet One® Swiss Sweet® Sunette®	This sweetener is heat stable and can be used in baking and cooking.
Sucralose	Splenda®	Sucralose is not affected by heat and retains sweetness in hot beverages, baked goods and processed foods.
Stevia	Truvia™	Stevia powder is 100% natural; ¾ teaspoon (one 3.5g packet) is equal in sweetness to 2 teaspoons sugar. Contact the manufacturer for recommended use of stevia in baking and cooking.

Vegetables

There are basically two types of vegetables – starchy and nonstarchy. Nonstarchy can be eaten in abundance, but starchy have more sugar, and portion sizes need to be kept in check. Nonstarchy vegetables include artichokes, asparagus, beets, broccoli, carrots, cauliflower, cucumber, eggplant, mushrooms, okra, onions, peppers, salad greens, spinach, tomatoes and zucchini. These vegetables form the basis of many of the recipes. Starchy vegetables include corn, peas, potatoes and squash, and are used in moderation.

Frozen vegetables and vegetable blends are frequently used in the recipes. Frozen "seasoning blend" is a mixture of chopped onions, celery, bell peppers and parsley. Other combinations include frozen pepper and onion strips, and stew and soup vegetables. It is not always necessary to thaw the vegetables before using in some recipes, especially soups and stews. It's even better to substitute fresh vegetables, just make changes in the recipes as needed.

Look for "Sally's Seasoning Blend," p. 217, which is minced garlic and chopped onions, celery and bell peppers. Fresh, not purchased, minced garlic is used in many recipes. Use a garlic press for most convenience in preparing garlic.

Most of the recipes specify no-salt or reduced-sodium canned vegetables. If using canned vegetables with sodium, drain the vegetables and rinse twice in water to cut back on sodium. Take advantage of the no-salt canned tomatoes, tomato sauce and tomato paste with additions of garlic, onion, basil, oregano and other seasonings.

What is the portion size of vegetables? A serving is ½ cup cooked and 1 cup raw.

A good rule of thumb in choosing vegetables is to eat a variety of colors. Choose dark green and deep yellow vegetables most often, such as zucchini.

References

American Diabetic Association. www.diabetes.org

American Dietetic Association. www.eatright.org

American Heart Association. www.amerianheart.org

Department of Agriculture (USDA). www.usda.gov

Food and Drug Administration (FDA). www.fda.gov

U.S. Food and Drug Administration, National Nutrient Database. www.nal.usda.gov-fnic

U.S. Food and Drug Administration, Center for Food Safety and Applied Nutrition. www.cfsan.fda.gov

Whitney, E. N. & S. R. Rolfes. *Understanding Nutrition*, 12th ed., 2011. Wadsworth, Cengage Learning.

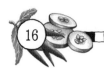

Food and Drug Administration (FDA) Nutrition Labeling

Nutrition Facts Label

If you learn to use the Nutrition Facts label, you will have an excellent source of knowledge to help you plan your daily food intake. It may take some practice to learn how to use the label effectively, but it will be worth it

The circled numbers by the below example of a Nutrition Facts label refer to the numbers shown with each explanation.

① Serving Size

Serving sizes are given in familiar units such as cups or pieces and also in metric measures. *See Nutrition Label at right. Example:* Serving Size 1 cup (266g).

② Servings Per Container

The label states how many servings of the food are in the package so you can plan how to use the food in a recipe or how much of the product you need to purchase.

See Nutrition Label at right. Example: Servings Per Container about 2.

Nutrition Facts		
① Serving Size 1 cup (266 g)		
② Servings Per Container about 2		
③ **Amount Per Serving**		
④ **Calories** 130 Calories from Fat 20 ⑤		
		% Daily Value* ⑥
⑦ **Total Fat** 2g		3%
Saturated Fat 1g		
Trans Fat 0g		
⑧ **Cholesterol** 10mg		9%
⑨ **Sodium** 890mg		37%
⑩ **Total Carbohydrate** 19g		6%
⑪ Dietary Fiber 4g		16%
⑫ Sugars 4g		
⑬ **Protein** 8g		
⑭ Vitamin A 60% • Vitamin C 2%		
Calcium 2% • Iron 6%		
⑮ *Percent Daily Values are based on a 2,000 calorie diet. Your daily values may be higher or lower depending on your calorie needs.		

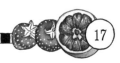
③ Amount Per Serving

This headline alerts you to the nutrient values in a single serving of the food. *See Nutrition Label, page 16.*

④ Calories

Calories are a measure of food energy or how much fuel your body can utilize from a single serving of the food. Many of us consume more calories than we need without getting the nutrients our bodies actually need. *See Nutrition Label, page 16. Example:* **Calories** 130.

⑤ Calories from Fat

This tells you how many of the total calories are from fat. *See Nutrition Label, page 16. Example:* Calories from Fat 20.

⑥ Percent (%) Daily Value

The percentages on the right side of the label refer to a standard Percent Daily Value based on a 2,000 calorie diet. Your Daily Value may be higher or lower depending on your individual calorie needs. *See Nutrition Label, page 16. Example: Total Fat 2g is 3% of the recommended % Daily Value for fat.*

⑦ Total Fat

Total Fat, measured in grams, includes grams of saturated fat and *trans* fat. This information is of particular interest to people concerned about high blood cholesterol and heart disease. *See Nutrition Label, page 16. Example:* **Total Fat** 2g.

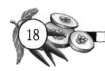

⑧ Cholesterol

Cholesterol is measured in milligrams (mg). Health experts recommend adults reduce cholesterol intake to less than 300 milligrams daily.

To maintain a healthy cholesterol intake, these recipes use liquid egg substitute and products that are reduced-fat or fat-free.

See Nutrition Label, page 16. Example: **Cholesterol** 10mg.

⑨ Sodium

Sodium is measured in milligrams (mg). Since our diets rarely lack sodium, sodium recommendations are set low enough to protect against high blood pressure and high enough to provide an adequate amount. The Daily Value used on food labels for sodium is 2,400 milligrams, however, health experts recommend that diabetics limit daily sodium intake to 2,300 milligrams per day. Only 1 teaspoon (5 grams) of salt contributes 2,000 milligrams sodium to the body.

Salt is NOT used as an ingredient in the recipes. High amounts of sodium are in many of our foods. As compared to fresh and frozen foods, processed foods (such as snack foods) contain the most sodium. *See Nutrition Label, page 16. Example:* **Sodium** 890mg.

⑩ Total Carbohydrate

Dietary recommendations are that carbohydrates should provide more than half of our daily energy (calories) intake. A variety of whole grains, vegetables, fruits and legumes (dried beans and peas) should be chosen daily.

The recipes include whole grain products, whole wheat breads, whole wheat tortillas, whole wheat pasta and brown rice in addition to a wide selection of fresh vegetables and fruits. Choose low-carb and reduced-fat products if they are available.

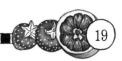
Carbohydrate is measured in grams (g). *See Nutrition Label, page 16.* *Example:* **Total Carbohydrate** 19g.

⑪ Dietary Fiber

The FDA recommends healthy adults consume 25 grams of dietary fiber daily. Dietary Fiber is measured in grams (g). Note that the grams of Total Carbohydrate on the label **include** the grams of fiber. *See Nutrition Label, page 16. Example:* Dietary Fiber 4g.

Where to get more fiber? Whole-grain products provide about 1 to 2 grams (or more) of fiber per serving, such as 1 slice whole wheat bread.

Most vegetables contain about 2 to 3 grams of fiber per ½ cup serving of cooked vegetable. Fresh fruits have about 2 grams of fiber per serving, such as 1 medium apple. About 8 grams of fiber are provided in ½ cup of cooked beans.

⑫ Sugars

According to experts, added sugars should contribute only 10 percent of energy intake (calories) per day. Foods that contain added sugar (cookies, cakes, sodas, etc.) generally contain lots of calories, but very few needed nutrients.

Fortunately, sugar substitutes are widely available today for use by individuals who desire sweetness in foods, without the added calories of sugar and other sweeteners. The recipes in this book generally use sugar substitutes instead of sugar.

Sugars are measured in grams (g). Note that the grams of Total Carbohydrate on the label **include** the grams of sugar. *See Nutrition Label, page 16. Example:* Sugars 4g.

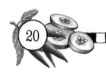

⑬ Protein

These recipes include a variety of protein sources that are low in fat and calories. On the Nutrition Facts label, the amount of protein in a single serving of food is given in grams. *See Nutrition Label, page 16.* *Example:* **Protein** 8g.

⑭ Additional Information

Most labels also include information about some of the vitamins and minerals in the food. *See Nutrition Label, page 16.*

⑮ Standard 2,000 Calorie Diet

Nutrition labels include a note of explanation that the Nutrition Facts are based on the FDA standard of a 2,000 calorie diet. Some labels also include information for a 2,500 calorie diet.

See Nutrition Label, page 16. Your personal calorie needs as determined by a health professional may be different from the FDA's standard used for Nutrition Facts labels.

Sources:

American Dietetic Association.   www.ada.org

U.S. Food and Drug Administration, Center for Food Safety and Applied Nutrition.   www.cfsan.fda.gov

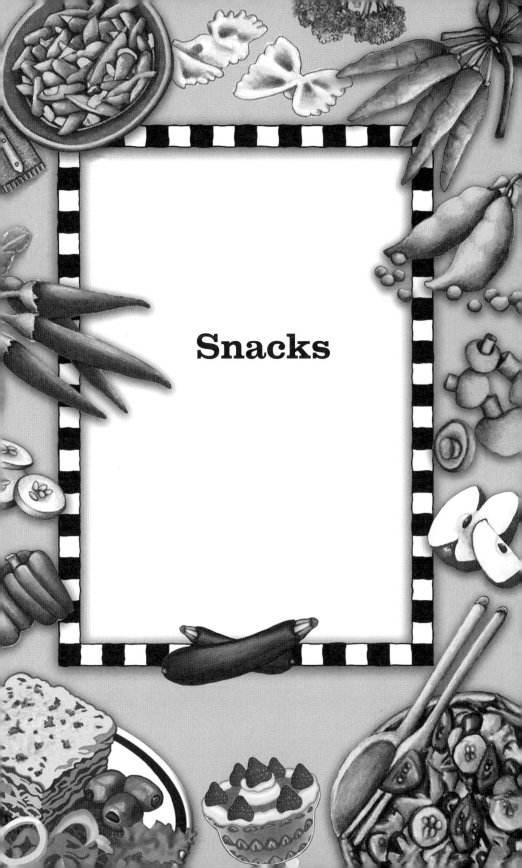

Snacks

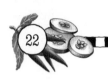

About Snacks

S nacking between meals is a good way to manage blood glucose
levels and spread calories and carbohydrates throughout the day.
Consider your overall food plan when choosing snacks. Also, snacking
between meals is not for everyone. Consult your nutritionist to
determine the best plan for you.

Snack Contents

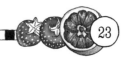

Tomato-Cheese Snack

1-inch cube reduced-fat colby-Jack cheese
1 cup cherry tomatoes

Quick Nutrition Facts
One Serving
Calories 142
Fat 9g
Carbohydrate 7g
Protein 8g

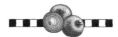

Cream Cheese-Melba Toast Snack

2 tablespoons reduced-fat cream cheese
4 whole grain melba toast rounds

Quick Nutrition Facts
One Serving
Calories 120
Fat 7g
Carbohydrate 10g
Protein 4g

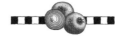

Cheese & Apple Snack

1 Mozzarella string cheese stick, 2% milk
1 small apple

Quick Nutrition Facts
One Serving
Calories 127
Fat 3g
Carbohydrate 21g
Protein 5g

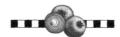

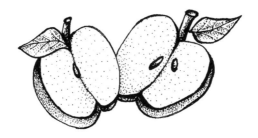

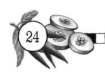

Mini-Taco Snack

1 small corn tostada shell
2 tablespoons bean dip
2 tablespoons fat-free shredded cheddar cheese

Quick Nutrition Facts	
One Serving	
Calories	108
Fat	3g
Carbohydrate	11g
Protein	8g

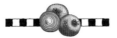

Dippin' Zucchini Snack

1 cup zucchini slices
¼ cup "Parmesan Ranch Dip," p. 41

Quick Nutrition Facts	
One Serving	
Calories	163
Fat	12g
Carbohydrate	10g
Protein	2g

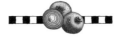

Rice Cake & Peanut Butter Snack

1 brown rice cake
1 tablespoon reduced-fat peanut butter

Quick Nutrition Facts	
One Serving	
Calories	115
Fat	6g
Carbohydrate	15g
Protein	5g

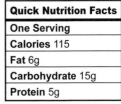

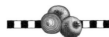

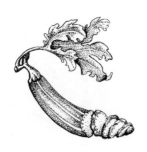

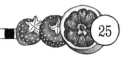

Milk & Grahams Snack

1 cup fat-free milk
2 reduced-fat graham cracker squares

Quick Nutrition Facts	
One Serving	
Calories	150
Fat	1g
Carbohydrate	25g
Protein	10g

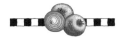

Blueberries with Yogurt Snack

6 ounces fat-free plain yogurt
½ cup blueberries

Quick Nutrition Facts	
One Serving	
Calories	122
Fat	0g
Carbohydrate	22g
Protein	8g

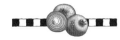

Strawberry Bagel Snack

½ small bagel
1 tablespoon reduced-fat cream cheese
1 tablespoon sugar-free strawberry preserves

Quick Nutrition Facts	
One Serving	
Calories	97
Fat	6g
Carbohydrate	18g
Protein	8g

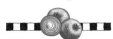

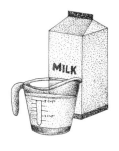

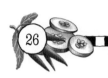

Veggie Juice & Popcorn Snack

1 cup reduced-sodium vegetable juice
3 cups microwave 94% fat-free popcorn

Quick Nutrition Facts
One Serving
Calories 100
Fat 1g
Carbohydrate 22g
Protein 4g

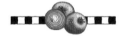

Almonds & Slaw Snack

½ cup "Three Green Slaw," p. 80
1 tablespoon whole natural almonds (14)

Quick Nutrition Facts
One Serving
Calories 149
Fat 9g
Carbohydrate 14g
Protein 6g

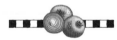

Cocoa & Crackers Snack

1 cup "Sugar-Free Hot Cocoa Mix," p. 62
10 mini saltine crackers

Quick Nutrition Facts
One Serving
Calories 112
Fat 1g
Carbohydrate 21g
Protein 8g

"Let food be thy medicine and medicine be thy food."

—Hippocrates

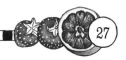

Cheese & Tomato Soup Snack

1 cup "Zesty Tomato Soup," p. 146
1-inch cube reduced-fat Colby-Jack cheese

Quick Nutrition Facts
One Serving
Calories 161
Fat 9g
Carbohydrate 10g
Protein 8g

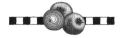

Bell Peppers & Salsa Snack

2 tablespoons "Corn and Black Bean
   Salsa," p. 57
1 cup red and yellow bell pepper strips

Quick Nutrition Facts
One Serving
Calories 53
Fat 0g
Carbohydrate 11g
Protein 3g

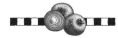

Broccoli with Dip Snack

1 cup broccoli florets
¼ cup "Quick Hummus," p. 44

Quick Nutrition Facts
One Serving
Calories 107
Fat 4g
Carbohydrate 14g
Protein 5g

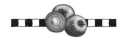

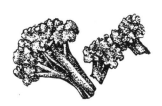

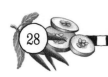

Fruit & Chocolate Yogo Pop Snack

1 (6 ounce) "Chocolate Yogo Pop," p. 243
½ small pear

Quick Nutrition Facts	
One Serving	
Calories 113	
Fat 0g	
Carbohydrate 26g	
Protein 3g	

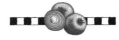

Grapes-Pistachio Snack

1 cup seedless grapes
1 tablespoon dry roasted pistachios

Quick Nutrition Facts	
One Serving	
Calories 97	
Fat 7g	
Carbohydrate 19g	
Protein 4g	

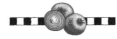

Slaw with Crackers Snack

¾ cup "Potluck Apple-Cabbage Mix-Up," p. 82
2 flatbread crackers

Quick Nutrition Facts	
One Serving	
Calories 124	
Fat 6g	
Carbohydrate 10g	
Protein 2g	

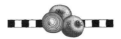

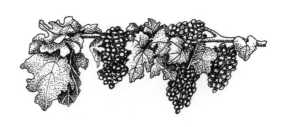

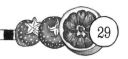

Pretzels & Cauliflower Snack

1 mini bag (17) tiny pretzel twists
1 cup cauliflower florets

Quick Nutrition Facts
One Serving
Calories 137
Fat 1g
Carbohydrate 28g
Protein 4g

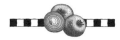

Snow Peas & Dip Snack

½ cup fresh snow peas
2 tablespoons "Dilly Dilly Dip," p. 36

Quick Nutrition Facts
One Serving
Calories 93
Fat 3g
Carbohydrate 5g
Protein 1g

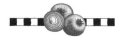

Guacamole-Carrots Snack

¼ cup "Green Green Guacamole," p. 38
1 cup baby carrots

Quick Nutrition Facts
One Serving
Calories 131
Fat 7g
Carbohydrate 16g
Protein 2g

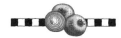

To help reduce high blood pressure, reduce and monitor your sodium intake.

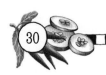

Pineapple-Cheese Treat Snack

½ cup reduced-fat cottage cheese
½ cup pineapple tidbits in juice

Quick Nutrition Facts
One Serving
Calories 140
Fat 2g
Carbohydrate 19g
Protein 12

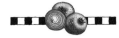

Gelatin with Topping Snack

1 (3 ounce) sugar-free gelatin snack cup
2 tablespoons reduced-fat whipped topping

Quick Nutrition Facts
One Serving
Calories 30
Fat 1g
Carbohydrate 3g
Protein 1g

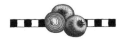

Spinach-Pepperoni Snack

1 cup spinach leaves
½ cup sliced mushrooms
1 tablespoon turkey pepperoni minis
1 tablespoon fat-free balsamic vinaigrette

Quick Nutrition Facts
One Serving
Calories 60
Fat 2g
Carbohydrate 8g
Protein 7g

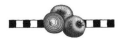

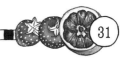

Banana-Yogurt Snack

½ banana
½ cup organic Greek yogurt

Quick Nutrition Facts	
One Serving	
Calories 162	
Fat 0g	
Carbohydrate 26g	
Protein 12g	

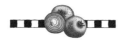

Orange & Milk Snack

1 small orange
1 cup reduced-fat vanilla soy milk

Quick Nutrition Facts	
One Serving	
Calories 125	
Fat 2g	
Carbohydrate 21g	
Protein 7g	

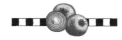

Tuna-Veggie Snack

¼ cup white albacore tuna
2 teaspoons lemon juice
1 cup baby greens
½ cup celery sticks

Quick Nutrition Facts	
One Serving	
Calories 99	
Fat 2g	
Carbohydrate 4g	
Protein 19g	

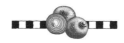

Chicken Soup & Tomatoes Snack

1 cup "Chicken Noodle Soup," p. 162
½ cup sliced tomatoes

Quick Nutrition Facts	
One Serving	
Calories 124	
Fat 2g	
Carbohydrate 18g	
Protein 11g	

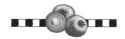

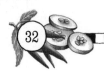

Mini Ham Sandwich Snack

1 slice "light style" wheat bread
1 ounce ultra-thin deli ham
1 slice fat-free cheese
1 teaspoon dijon-style mustard

Quick Nutrition Facts
One Serving
Calories 100
Fat 1g
Carbohydrate 13g
Protein 10g

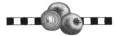

Melon & Rice Cake Snack

1 cup "Icy Cantaloupe Crush," p. 63
1 brown rice cake

Quick Nutrition Facts
One Serving
Calories 91
Fat 0g
Carbohydrate 20g
Protein 2g

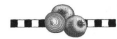

Milk & O's Snack

1 cup doughnut-shaped oat cereal
½ cup fat-free milk

Quick Nutrition Facts
One Serving
Calories 145
Fat 2g
Carbohydrate 26
Protein 8g

Weight Management: Eat slowly.

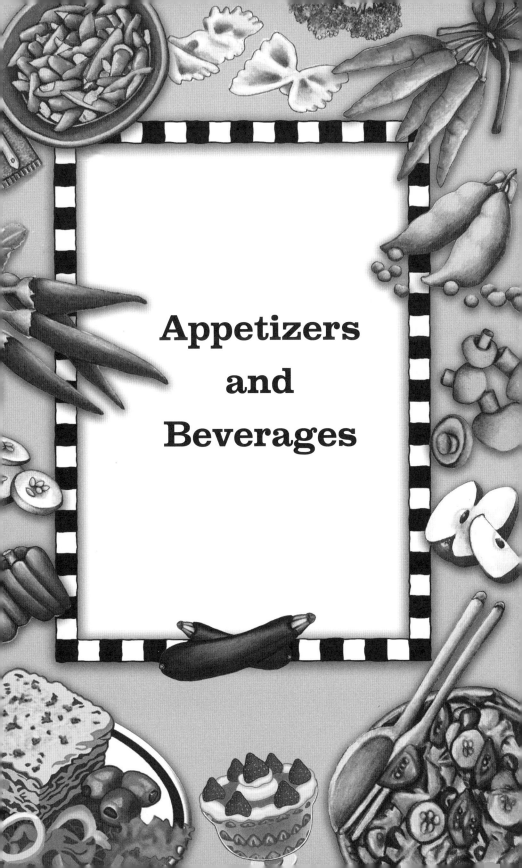

Appetizers
and
Beverages

Appetizers and Beverages Contents

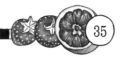

Crunchy Zucchini Slices

2 medium zucchini, cut in ¾-inch thick
    bias slices
¼ cup panko (Japanese-style) breadcrumbs
1 tablespoon grated parmesan cheese
1 tablespoon reduced-fat mayonnaise

Nutrition Facts		
Serving Size 2 slices		
Servings Per Recipe 6		
Amount Per Serving		
Calories 28		
Total Fat 1g		
Cholesterol 2mg		
Sodium 41mg		
Total Carbohydrate 3g		
Dietary Fiber 1g		
Sugars 2g		
Protein 1g		

1. In medium saucepan, heat 1 inch water until it boils.

2. Add zucchini slices, reduce heat and simmer for 3 to 5 minutes, until just tender. Drain and pat dry with paper towels.

3. Preheat broiler. Mix crumbs and cheese. Spread mayonnaise on one side of each zucchini slice.

4. Coat that side with crumbs and arrange on foil-lined baking sheet. Broil 4 to 5 inches from heat for 2 to 3 minutes.

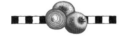

Spray a grater with nonstick cooking spray before grating cheese and cleanup will be a snap.

Curried Deviled Eggs

8 hard-cooked eggs
¼ cup reduced-fat mayonnaise
2 teaspoons dijon-style mustard
¼ teaspoon curry powder

1. Halve eggs lengthwise and remove yolks. Mash egg yolks and mix with remaining ingredients.

2. Whisk until smooth and spoon on egg white halves. Cover and refrigerate.

Nutrition Facts
Serving Size 1 half egg
Servings Per Recipe 16
Amount Per Serving
Calories 48
Total Fat 3g
Cholesterol 107mg
Sodium 50mg
Total Carbohydrate 1g
Dietary Fiber 0g
Sugars 0g
Protein 3g

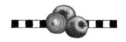

Dilly Dilly Dip

½ cup reduced-fat mayonnaise
½ cup reduced-fat sour cream
1 teaspoon lemon juice
1 teaspoon dried dill weed

1. Mix ingredients. Cover and refrigerate. Makes 1 cup.

Nutrition Facts
Serving Size 2 tablespoons
Servings Per Recipe 8
Amount Per Serving
Calories 80
Total Fat 6g
Cholesterol 19mg
Sodium 34mg
Total Carbohydrate 4g
Dietary Fiber 0g
Sugars 3g
Protein 1g

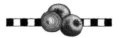

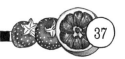

Fresh Salsa Verde

6 - 8 medium fresh tomatillos, husked,
    stemmed, chopped*
2 medium jalapeño peppers, seeded, finely
    chopped
3 tablespoons finely chopped red onion
¼ cup chopped cilantro

1. Stir ingredients together. Cover and
    refrigerate 4 hours before serving.

*TIP: Small, green tomatoes will substitute for
    fresh tomatillos.*

Nutrition Facts		
Serving Size ¼ cup		
Servings Per Recipe 10		
Amount Per Serving		
Calories 9		
Total Fat 0g		
Cholesterol 0mg		
Sodium 0mg		
Total Carbohydrate 2g		
Dietary Fiber 1g		
Sugars 1g		
Protein 0g		

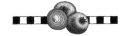

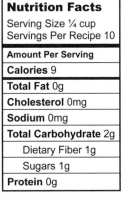

Tomatillos, used in Mexican dishes, resemble a
small, green tomato and have a papery husk. You
will generally find fresh tomatillos in specialty
produce markets. If not fresh, you can find
tomatillos canned in water and also in green salsas.

Hearty Red Pepper Spread

1 (8 ounce) package reduced-fat cream cheese
⅓ cup chopped roasted red pepper
1 teaspoon dried basil, crushed
½ teaspoon garlic powder

1. Mix ingredients and refrigerate.

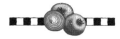

Nutrition Facts
Serving Size 2 tablespoons
Servings Per Recipe 8
Amount Per Serving
Calories 34
Total Fat 2g
Cholesterol 0mg
Sodium 71mg
Total Carbohydrate 2g
Dietary Fiber 0g
Sugars 1g
Protein 1g

Green Green Guacamole

2 ripe Hass avocados
2 tablespoons finely chopped canned
    green chilies
1 teaspoon finely chopped green onion
2 teaspoons lime juice

1. Halve avocados, remove seeds, peel and
slightly mash. Mix with remaining
ingredients. Cover and refrigerate.
Makes 2 cups.

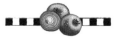

Nutrition Facts
Serving Size ¼ cup
Servings Per Recipe 8
Amount Per Serving
Calories 81
Total Fat 7g
Cholesterol 0mg
Sodium 6mg
Total Carbohydrate 4g
Dietary Fiber 3g
Sugars 0g
Protein 1g

The tradition of providing British sailors with citrus juice daily to prevent scurvy gave them the nickname "limeys."

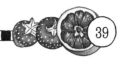
Hot Artichoke Dip

1 (8 ounce) can artichoke hearts in water,
    drained, coarsely chopped
¼ cup finely grated jalapeño pepper-Jack
    cheese
¾ cup reduced-fat mayonnaise
1 teaspoon lemon juice

1. Preheat oven to 350°.

2. Mix ingredients and spread in ungreased
    1 to 1½ -quart shallow baking dish.

3. Bake 20 to 30 minutes or until it bubbles.
    Serve warm or cold.

Nutrition Facts	
Serving Size 2 tablespoons Servings Per Recipe 16	
Amount Per Serving	
Calories 34	
Total Fat 2g	
Cholesterol 3mg	
Sodium 90mg	
Total Carbohydrate 2g	
Dietary Fiber 0g	
Sugars 1g	
Protein 1g	

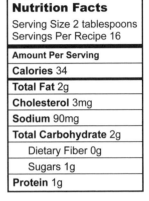

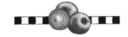

*When a recipe calls for artichoke hearts, use
frozen or canned in water. Otherwise, artichokes
canned in an oil-based marinade will be specified.*

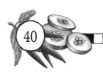

Mozzarella-Tomato Bruschetta

8 (½ inch) slices baguette-style bread
4 medium Roma tomatoes, seeded, chopped
¼ teaspoon dried oregano, crushed
2 ounces finely shredded reduced-fat
    mozzarella cheese

Nutrition Facts		
Serving size 1 bruschetta Servings Per Recipe 8		
Amount Per Serving		
Calories 42		
Total Fat 1g		
Cholesterol 5mg		
Sodium 78mg		
Total Carbohydrate 5g		
Dietary Fiber 0g		
Sugars 1g		
Protein 3g		

1. Preheat oven to 350°.

2. Arrange bread slices on baking sheet and spray one side. Bake 3 to 4 minutes or until lightly toasted.

3. Stir together tomatoes and oregano and spoon onto untoasted side of bread.

4. Sprinkle with cheese and bake just until cheese melts.

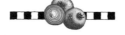

Did you know that grape tomatoes are baby Romas?

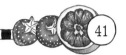
Parmesan Ranch Dip

½ cup fat-free ranch-style salad dressing
½ cup reduced-fat mayonnaise
½ cup reduced-fat sour cream
⅓ cup grated parmesan cheese

1. Stir ingredients together. Cover and refrigerate 1 to 2 hours. Makes 1½ cups.

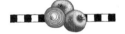

Nutrition Facts
Serving Size 2 tablespoons
Servings Per Recipe 12
Amount Per Serving
Calories 72
Total Fat 6g
Cholesterol 15mg
Sodium 115mg
Total Carbohydrate 3g
Dietary Fiber 0g
Sugars 2g
Protein 1g

There is a time every day when the phones go unanswered, the TV is off and e-mails can wait. For this short time, you are family and it is your dinnertime.

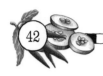

Pineapple Salsa

1 cup canned pineapple tidbits, coarsely
  chopped, drained
½ cup seeded, chopped Roma tomatoes
2 tablespoons snipped fresh cilantro
1 - 2 teaspoons finely chopped fresh jalapeño
  pepper

1. Stir ingredients together. Cover tightly and
   refrigerate.

Nutrition Facts	
Serving Size 2 tablespoons	
Servings Per Recipe 12	
Amount Per Serving	
Calories 35	
Total Fat 0g	
Cholesterol 0mg	
Sodium 1mg	
Total Carbohydrate 2g	
Dietary Fiber 0g	
Sugars 2g	
Protein 0g	

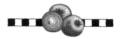

*Roma tomatoes, also called plum and Italian
plum, are a flavorful egg-shaped tomato, usually
less expensive than other types of tomatoes.*

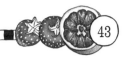
Quick Crab Appetizer

1 (3 ounce) package reduced-fat cream cheese
1 (6 ounce) can minced white crab, drained
¾ cup "Seafood Cocktail Sauce," p. 218
1 tablespoon chopped parsley for garnish

1. Place cream cheese on small serving dish.

2. In small bowl, mix crab and seafood sauce. Spoon onto cream cheese and garnish with parsley.

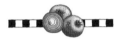

Nutrition Facts		
Serving Size 2 tablespoons		
Servings Per Recipe 14		
Amount Per Serving		
Calories 37		
Total Fat 2g		
Cholesterol 16mg		
Sodium 203mg		
Total Carbohydrate 2g		
Dietary Fiber 2g		
Sugars 0g		
Protein 2g		

An appetizer is described as any small, bite-size food served before a meal to whet and excite the palate. The term also applies to a first course served at table.

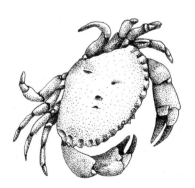

Quick Hummus

1 (15 ounce) can garbanzo beans, drained,
     liquid reserved
2 teaspoons minced garlic
2 tablespoons fresh lemon juice
2 tablespoons olive oil

1. In blender or food processor, process
ingredients about 30 seconds. Add reserved
bean liquid until of desired consistency.

Nutrition Facts	
Serving Size ¼ cup	
Servings Per Recipe 8	
Amount Per Serving	
Calories 76	
Total Fat 4g	
Cholesterol 0mg	
Sodium 123mg	
Total Carbohydrate 8g	
Dietary Fiber 2g	
Sugars 1g	
Protein 2g	

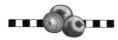

Garbanzo beans, also known as chick peas, are a healthy addition to salads, soups and stews.

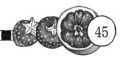

Red and Green Salsa

2 cups seeded, chopped Roma tomatoes
¼ cup finely chopped onion
1 (4 ounce) can diced green chilies, drained,
    liquid reserved
1 tablespoon fresh lime juice

1. Mix ingredients. Add small amount of
   reserved liquid until of desired consistency.

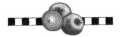

Nutrition Facts	
Serving Size 2 tablespoons	
Servings Per Recipe 20	
Amount Per Serving	
Calories 5	
Total Fat 0g	
Cholesterol 0mg	
Sodium 5mg	
Total Carbohydrate 1g	
Dietary Fiber 0g	
Sugars 1g	
Protein 0g	

Salsa, the Spanish word for sauce, can range in spiciness from mild to very hot and can be cooked or uncooked. Salsa cruda refers to an uncooked salsa."

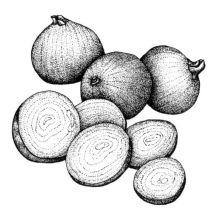

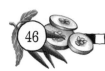

Roasted Zucchini Dip

3 medium zucchini, sliced
1 medium red bell pepper, sliced
1 medium red onion, sliced
2 cloves garlic, peeled

1. Preheat oven to 400°.

2. Spread vegetables on sprayed foil-lined baking pan. Bake 15 minutes and stir.

3. Spray and bake additional 15 minutes or until vegetables are tender.

4. Transfer to blender or food processor. Cover and process 30 to 60 seconds. Serve warm or cold.

Nutrition Facts		
Serving size ¼ cup		
Servings Per recipe 16		
Amount Per Serving		
Calories 14		
Total Fat 0g		
Cholesterol 0mg		
Sodium 3mg		
Total Carbohydrate 3g		
Dietary Fiber 1g		
Sugars 2g		
Protein 1g		

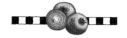

Do you know why New Englanders have to lock their cars in September? To keep the seats from being filled with zucchini!

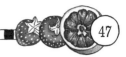

Teriyaki Pork Meatballs

1 pound lean ground pork
⅓ cup finely chopped green onion
¼ cup soft light-style wheat breadcrumbs
⅓ cup reduced-sodium teriyaki marinade,
    divided

Nutrition Facts	
Serving Size 2 meatballs	
Servings Per Recipe 10	
Amount Per Serving	
Calories 110	
Total Fat 7g	
Cholesterol 31mg	
Sodium 195mg	
Total Carbohydrate 2g	
Dietary Fiber 0g	
Sugars 2g	
Protein 9g	

1. Preheat oven to 425°.

2. Mix pork, onions, breadcrumbs and
   2 tablespoons marinade.

3. Use 2 tablespoons mixture to make about
   20 meatballs.

4. Arrange meatballs on sprayed foil-lined baking pan. Brush
   meatballs with marinade.

5. Bake 15 minutes or until no longer pink; baste once or twice.

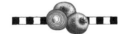

Today's pork is leaner (about one-third fewer calories) and higher in protein than pork available to consumers just 10 years ago.

Toasty Asparagus Rolls

10 - 15 fresh asparagus spears, trimmed
10 slices light-style wheat bread, crusts
   trimmed
1½ tablespoons reduced-fat mayonnaise
5 reduced-fat mozzarella cheese sticks,
   pulled apart

Nutrition Facts	
Serving Size 1 roll	
Servings Per Recipe 10	
Amount Per Serving	
Calories 80	
Total Fat 3g	
Cholesterol 8mg	
Sodium 208mg	
Total Carbohydrate 10g	
Dietary Fiber 3g	
Sugars 1g	
Protein 7g	

1. In 10 to 12-inch skillet, heat 1 inch water until it boils.

2. Add asparagus, cover and cook 7 to 10 minutes, until just tender. Drain.

3. With rolling pin, slightly flatten each bread slice. Spread 1 teaspoon mayonnaise on one side bread.

4. Top that side with 1 to 2 asparagus spears and 3 to 4 cheese strings. Roll carefully.

5. Preheat broiler. On sprayed baking sheet, arrange rolls seam side down and spray again.

6. Broil 4 to 5 inches from heat for 3 to 5 minutes or until bread browns.

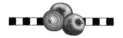

To revive limp asparagus, cut off ¼-inch of the stem ends, stand the spears vertically in about 2 inches ice water. Cover with a plastic bag and refrigerate about 2 hours.

Veggie Pizza Snack

2 (6 inch) pita breads
¾ cup assorted fresh vegetables (mushrooms,
    bell pepper, carrots, broccoli)
⅓ cup pizza sauce
¼ cup shredded reduced fat mozzarella cheese

1. Preheat oven to 400°.

2. Do not split pita breads. Bake breads for
3 to 4 minutes.

3. Add assorted vegetables to sprayed nonstick
6 to 8-inch skillet over medium heat. Cook
and stir until just tender.

4. Spread pizza sauce on pita bread. Sprinkle with vegetables and
cheese and bake 10 minutes or until light brown. Cut in half
to serve.

Nutrition Facts
Serving Size ½ pita bread
Servings Per Recipe 4
Amount Per Serving
Calories 98
Total Fat 2g
Cholesterol 3mg
Sodium 263mg
Total Carbohydrate 14g
Dietary Fiber 1g
Sugars 2g
Protein 5g

*In 1938, a chemist named Roy Plunkett
inadvertently discovered Teflon – the essential
material in nonstick cookware today, making it
easy to cook food without fat.*

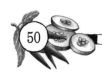

Apple-Feta Crostini

16 (½-inch) slices baguette-style bread
½ cup crumbled reduced-fat feta cheese
1 medium apple, halved, cored, thinly sliced
2 tablespoons honey

Nutrition Facts	
Serving Size 2 crostini	
Servings Per Recipe 8	
Amount Per Serving	
Calories 103	
Total Fat 3g	
Cholesterol 13mg	
Sodium 224mg	
Total Carbohydrate 16g	
Dietary Fiber 1g	
Sugars 7 g	
Protein 4g	

1. Arrange bread slices on large baking sheet. Broil 4 to 5 inches from heat for 30 to 60 seconds.

2. Turn bread slices over and top with feta cheese. Broil 30 to 60 seconds or until cheese bubbles.

3. Top bread slices with apple slices and drizzle with honey.

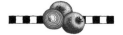

Avocado-Seafood Dip

1 (6 ounce) can solid white albacore tuna
   in water
2 large Hass avocados, pitted, peeled, slightly
   mashed
2 tablespoons fresh lemon juice
3 teaspoons prepared horseradish

Nutrition Facts	
Serving Size ¼ cup	
Servings Per Recipe 10	
Amount Per Serving	
Calories: 85	
Total Fat 6g	
Cholesterol 5mg	
Sodium 65mg	
Total Carbohydrate 4g	
Dietary Fiber 3g	
Sugars 0g	
Protein 5g	

1. Drain and flake tuna. Mix with avocado, lemon juice and horseradish. Cover and refrigerate. Makes 2½ cups.

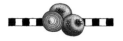

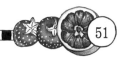

Barbecued Chicken Wings

1 pound (about 8) chicken wing drumettes,
   trimmed
½ cup "Low-Carb Barbecue Sauce, " p. 223

Nutrition Facts	
Serving Size 2 wings	
Servings Per Recipe 4	
Amount Per Serving	
Calories 118	
Total Fat 8g	
Cholesterol 40mg	
Sodium 321mg	
Total Carbohydrate 4g	
Dietary Fiber 0g	
Sugars 8g	
Protein 9g	

1. Preheat oven to 350°.

2. Rinse wings and pat dry with paper towels.
    Dip wings in sauce and place on sprayed foil-
    lined baking sheet.

3. Brush with barbecue sauce and bake
    uncovered for 30 to 40 minutes; baste
    occasionally.

4. Turn over, brush with sauce and bake additional 30 minutes or
    until tender.

*TIP: If you opt to buy barbecue sauce instead of making a barbecue sauce for
       this recipe, look for low-carb barbecue sauces now available.*

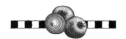

*Most adult females need around 1,600 calories
per day, whereas adult males need about 2,200
daily calories.*

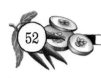

Black Bean Salsa

1 (15 ounce) can black beans, rinsed, drained
1 cup chopped fresh tomatoes with juice
⅓ cup finely chopped red onion
1 - 2 tablespoons snipped cilantro

1. Mash black beans, but leave chunks. Stir together black beans, tomatoes and onion.

2. Top with cilantro. Cover and refrigerate.

Nutrition Facts	
Serving Size ¼ cup	
Servings Per Recipe 10	
Amount Per Serving	
Calories 18	
Total Fat 0g	
Cholesterol 0mg	
Sodium 41mg	
Total Carbohydrate 3g	
Dietary Fiber 1g	
Sugars 1g	
Protein 1g	

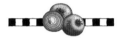

When using canned beans and peas, my rule of thumb is to rinse twice and drain to freshen and remove additives in the liquid (unless the liquid is used in the recipe.)

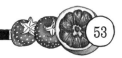
Broiled Vegetable Antipasto

1 medium red bell pepper
10 - 12 thin fresh asparagus spears, trimmed
1½ cups fresh small white mushrooms,
    cleaned, halved
2 tablespoons balsamic vinegar

Nutrition Facts		
Serving Size ½ cup		
Servings Per Recipe 6		
Amount Per Serving		
Calories 20		
Total Fat 0g		
Cholesterol 0mg		
Sodium 3mg		
Total Carbohydrate 4g		
Dietary Fiber 1g		
Sugars 2g		
Protein 1g		

1. Preheat broiler.

2. On foil-lined baking sheet, broil red pepper,
   4 to 5 inches from heat, on all sides until
   charred.

3. Remove and seal in plastic bag until cool
   enough to handle.

4. Under cold running water, remove skin and seeds. Cut into
   ½-inch slices and place on serving dish.

5. Spread asparagus and mushrooms on foil-lined baking sheet
   and spray.

6. Broil, 4 to 5 inches from heat, turning frequently, until lightly
   browned.

7. Transfer asparagus and mushrooms to serving dish with bell pepper
   and drizzle with vinegar.

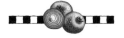

*Use a mushroom brush or damp paper towel to
clean mushrooms. If necessary to rinse them in
water, dry them quickly on paper towels before
they absorb too much moisture.*

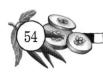

Cannellini Hummus with Pine Nuts

2 tablespoons pine nuts
1 cup canned cannellini beans, drained,
    liquid reserved
1 lemon
¼ teaspoon garlic powder

Nutrition Facts
Serving Size 2 tablespoons
Number of Servings 8
Amount Per Serving
Calories 37
Total Fat 1g
Cholesterol 0mg
Sodium 68mg
Total Carbohydrate 5g
Dietary Fiber 2g
Sugars 0g
Protein 2g

1. Toast pine nuts in dry skillet over low heat until light brown and fragrant.

2. Mash cannellini beans. Grate 1 teaspoon lemon peel and measure 1 to 2 tablespoons lemon juice.

3. Mix beans, lemon peel, lemon juice and garlic powder.

4. Stir in small amounts of reserved bean liquid until of desired consistency. Sprinkle with pine nuts.

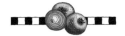

Store pine nuts in your freezer because they are high in fat and turn rancid easily.

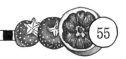

Cheese Stuffed Mushrooms

12 large fresh white mushrooms
½ cup finely chopped onion
¼ cup chopped ripe olives
2 - 3 tablespoons crumbled feta cheese

Nutrition Facts	
Serving Size 1 mushroom Servings Per Recipe 12	
Amount Per Serving	
Calories 15	
Total Fat 1g	
Cholesterol 1mg	
Sodium 43mg	
Total Carbohydrate 2g	
Dietary Fiber 0g	
Sugars 1g	
Protein 1g	

1. Preheat oven to 425°.

1. Remove stems from mushroom caps. Chop stems into small pieces.

2. Spray mushroom caps and arrange on foil-lined baking sheet. Bake for 5 minutes. Drain on paper towels.

3. In sprayed nonstick 10-inch skillet on medium heat, cook and stir mushroom stems and onion until tender.

4. Mix mushroom stems, onion, olives and cheese and spoon on mushroom caps. Bake 5 minutes or until hot and bubbly.

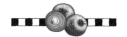

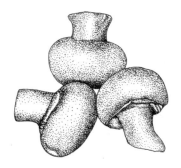

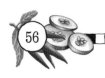

Cherry Tomatoes and Boursin Cheese

10 cherry tomatoes, halved
½ cup garlic-herb Boursin® cheese
Chopped parsley for garnish

1. Scoop seeds and flesh from tomato halves with small melon baller.

2. Spoon about 1 teaspoon cheese into tomato halves. Garnish with parsley.

Nutrition Facts	
Serving Size 2 tomato halves	
Servings Per Recipe 10	
Amount per Serving	
Calories 53	
Total Fat 5g	
Cholesterol 12mg	
Sodium 73mg	
Total Carbohydrate 2g	
Dietary Fiber 0g	
Sugars 1g	
Protein 1g	

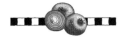

Boursin® cheese, usually found in deli sections, has a creamy, smooth texture and comes in many lively flavors. Look for light boursin to reduce calories and fat and still enjoy this delicious, appetizer cheese.

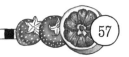
Citrus Shrimp Appetizer

1 (16 ounce) package frozen cooked large
   shrimp, peeled with tail, veined
¼ cup "Ginger-Orange Marinade," p. 225

1. Thaw frozen shrimp according to package directions. Drain on paper towels and place in resealable plastic bag.

2. Pour marinade over shrimp and seal bag. Refrigerate 1 to 2 hours. Drain and serve immediately.

Nutrition Facts	
Serving Size 2 shrimp Servings Per Recipe 6	
Amount Per Serving	
Calories 21	
Total Fat 0g	
Cholesterol 21mg	
Sodium 22mg	
Total Carbohydrate 2g	
Dietary Fiber 0g	
Sugars 1g	
Protein 3g	

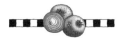

Corn and Black Bean Salsa

1 cup canned diced tomatoes and green chilies
1 cup black beans, drained, rinsed
1 cup frozen corn, cooked, drained
½ cup finely chopped onion

1. Process tomatoes and green chilies for 5 to 10 seconds in food processor or blender. Mix tomatoes with beans, corn and onion.

Nutrition Facts	
Serving size 2 tablespoons Servings per Recipe 12	
Amount per Serving	
Calories 35	
Total Fat 0g	
Cholesterol 0mg	
Sodium 81mg	
Total Carbohydrate 7g	
Dietary Fiber 2g	
Sugars 1g	
Protein 2g	

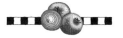

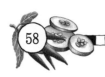

Cranberry Walnut Spread

1 (8 ounce) package reduced-fat cream cheese,
    softened
½ cup sweetened dried cranberries
3 teaspoons finely grated orange peel
¼ cup chopped toasted walnuts

1. Mix cream cheese, cranberries and orange
peel and refrigerate. Sprinkle with walnuts.

*TIP: To make this a 3-ingredient recipe, substitute
orange-flavor sweetened dried cranberries to
eliminate the freshly grated orange peel.*

Nutrition Facts
Serving Size 1 tablespoon
Servings Per Recipe 16
Amount Per Serving
Calories 54
Total Fat 3g
Cholesterol 8mg
Sodium 71mg
Total Carbohydrate 5g
Dietary Fiber 0g
Sugars 3g
Protein 1g

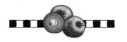

Creamy Fruit Dunk

1 (8 ounce) package reduced-fat cream
    cheese, softened
½ cup packed brown sugar-sugar substitute
    blend
2 tablespoons powdered sugar
1 teaspoon vanilla extract

1. Beat cream cheese and sugars until creamy.
Stir in vanilla.

Nutrition Facts
Serving Size 2 tablespoons
Servings Per Recipe 8
Amount Per Serving
Calories 74
Total Fat 2g
Cholesterol 8mg
Sodium 73mg
Total Carbohydrate 12g
Dietary Fiber 0g
Sugars 12g
Protein 1g

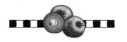

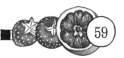
Crispy Chicken Bites

1 cup corn flake crumbs
½ cup reduced-fat baking mix
½ teaspoon paprika
2 medium boneless, skinless chicken breast
    halves, cut in 1-inch pieces

Nutrition Facts	
Serving Size 2 bites	
Servings Per Recipe 15	
Amount Per Serving	
Calories 34	
Total Fat 1g	
Cholesterol 3mg	
Sodium 81mg	
Total Carbohydrate 5g	
Dietary Fiber 0g	
Sugars 0g	
Protein 2g	

1. Preheat oven to 400°.

2. Mix crumbs, baking mix and paprika in large resealable plastic bag. Add half chicken pieces and shake to coat.

3. Arrange coated chicken pieces on foil-lined baking sheet and spray.

4. Bake 20 to 30 minutes or until chicken is no longer pink. Repeat with remaining chicken pieces.

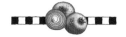

One sure way to tell if your fridge temperature is too warm is if milk sours before the sell-by date. It may be wise to check temperature with a thermometer and keep the fridge at 37°F.

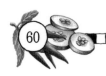

Coffee Deluxe

1 cup hot decaffeinated coffee
1 tablespoon sugar-free caramel syrup
1 tablespoon thawed reduced-fat frozen
    whipped topping

1. Pour coffee and syrup in large mug and stir. Top with whipped topping.

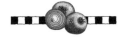

Nutrition Facts	
Serving Size 1 cup	
Servings Per Recipe 1	
Amount Per Serving	
Calories 55	
Total Fat 1g	
Cholesterol 0mg	
Sodium 41mg	
Total Carbohydrate 13g	
Dietary Fiber 0g	
Sugars 1g	
Protein 0g	

Snappy Ginger Tea

2 tablespoons lemon juice
1 tablespoon peeled finely grated ginger root
Sugar substitute equal to 2 - 3 teaspoons sugar

1. Combine lemon juice, ginger root and sugar substitute with 2 cups hot water. Stir well and let stand for 30 minutes.

2. Strain the mixture and pour into 2 glasses filled with ice.

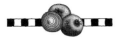

Nutrition Facts	
Serving Size 1 glass	
Servings Per Recipe 2	
Amount Per Serving	
Calories 7	
Total Fat 0g	
Cholesterol 0mg	
Sodium 1mg	
Total Carbohydrate 2g	
Dietary Fiber 0g	
Sugars 0g	
Protein 0g	

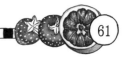

Green Tea Thirst Quencher

3 decaffeinated green tea bags
1 mint tea bag
1 (17 fluid ounce) bottle diet lemon-lime
  soda, cold

1. Pour 3 cups boiling water over tea bags.
    Cover and steep for 5 minutes. Remove tea
    bags and refrigerate tea until cold. Add soda
    and serve over ice.

Nutrition Facts	
Serving Size 1 cup Servings Per Recipe 5	
Amount Per Serving	
Calories 0	
Total Fat 0g	
Cholesterol 0mg	
Sodium 12mg	
Total Carbohydrate 0g	
Dietary Fiber 0g	
Sugars 0g	
Protein 0g	

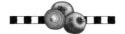

*Experts agree – drinking tea is healthy. Tea's
health benefits are mainly due to a high content
of flavonoids – plant-derived compounds that
are antioxidants.*

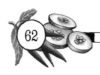

Sugar-Free Sports Drink

2 tablespoons lemon juice
Pinch salt
1 - 2 teaspoons sugar-free flavored drink mix

1. Mix all ingredients with 1 cup water and refrigerate.

Nutrition Facts	
Serving Size 1	
Servings per Recipe 1	
Amount Per Serving	
Calories 36	
Total Fat 0g	
Cholesterol 0mg	
Sodium 496mg	
Total Carbohydrate 14g	
Dietary Fiber 0g	
Sugars 0g	
Protein 0g	

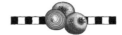

Sugar-Free Hot Cocoa Mix

3½ cups fat-free dry milk powder
Sugar substitute equal to 2 cups sugar
1 cup fat-free powdered nondairy creamer
½ cup unsweetened cocoa powder

1. Sift ingredients separately to remove lumps. Mix all ingredients in large bowl and store tightly covered.

2. To make one serving, spoon ⅓ cup cocoa mix in mug. Pour in ¾ cup boiling water and stir.

Nutrition Facts	
Serving Size ⅓ cup mix	
Servings Per Recipe 20	
Amount Per Serving	
Calories 108	
Total Fat 0g	
Cholesterol 4mg	
Sodium 124mg	
Total Carbohydrate 15g	
Dietary Fiber 0g	
Sugars 11g	
Protein 8g	

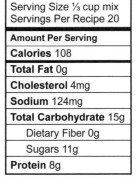

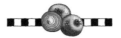

Weight Management: Limit concentrated sweets and alcoholic beverages.

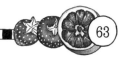
Icy Cantaloupe Crush

2 cups (1 inch) cubes cantaloupe
Sugar substitute equal to 4 teaspoons sugar
2 teaspoons lime juice

1. Place cantaloupe cubes in medium bowl.
   Stir sugar substitute and lime juice together
   and drizzle over cantaloupe. Toss to mix.

2. Pour cantaloupe and 1 cup crushed ice into
   blender and process just until smooth.

Nutrition Facts	
Serving size 1 cup	
Servings Per Recipe 2	
Amount Per Serving	
Calories 56	
Total Fat 0g	
Cholesterol 0mg	
Sodium 26mg	
Total Carbohydrate 13g	
Dietary Fiber 1g	
Sugars 13g	
Protein 1g	

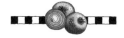

*According to a Harvard Medical School
publication, drinking a cup of freshly brewed
tea three times a day is the best way to get the
antioxidant benefits of green, black and oolong teas.*

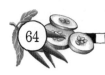

Cantaloupe Smoothie

1 cup (1 inch) cubes cantaloupe
½ cup fat-free organic vanilla Greek yogurt
¼ teaspoon lemon juice
Sugar substitute equal to 1 teaspoon sugar

1. Pulse ingredients in blender until smooth.

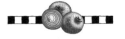

Nutrition Facts	
Serving Size 1 cup	
Servings Per Recipe 1	
Amount Per Serving	
Calories 134	
Total Fat 0g	
Cholesterol 0mg	
Sodium 71mg	
Total Carbohydrate 22g	
Dietary Fiber 1g	
Sugars 21g	
Protein 12g	

When using a food processor or blender, "pulsing" is a method of quick on/off pulses to keep pieces of food in the blade's path and from bouncing around the container. In the OFF position, use a wooden spoon handle to loosen food pieces from around a blender blade.

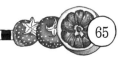

Best Strawberry Smoothie

1 cup fat-free milk
⅓ cup fat-free dry milk powder
1¼ cups frozen unsweetened whole
    strawberries
Sugar substitute equal to 2 teaspoons sugar

1. Process fat-free milk, dry milk and ½ cup
   water in blender about 15 seconds. Add
   strawberries and sugar substitute and pulse
   until smooth.

Nutrition Facts	
Serving Size 1 cup Servings Per Recipe 2	
Amount Per Serving	
Calories 114	
Total Fat 0g	
Cholesterol 4mg	
Sodium 128mg	
Total Carbohydrate 20g	
Dietary Fiber 2g	
Sugars 18g	
Protein 9g	

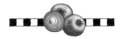

Pineapple-Blueberry Smoothie

1 (6 ounce) carton reduced-fat vanilla yogurt
1 cup fresh blueberries
½ cup canned crushed pineapple with juice

1. Place yogurt, blueberries, pineapple with
   juice and 1 cup crushed ice in blender
   or food processor. Process just until ice
   is blended.

Nutrition Facts	
Serving Size 1 cup Servings Per Recipe 3	
Amount Per Serving	
Calories 78	
Total Fat 0g	
Cholesterol 2mg	
Sodium 42mg	
Total Carbohydrate 18g	
Dietary Fiber 2g	
Sugars 13g	
Protein 3g	

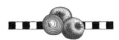

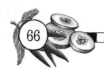

Orangesicle Smoothie

1 cup fat-free milk
⅓ cup fat-free dry milk powder
2 tablespoons frozen orange juice concentrate

1. Process milk, powder, orange juice concentrate and 1 cup crushed ice in blender until smooth.

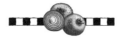

Nutrition Facts	
Serving Size 1 cup	
Servings Per Recipe 2	
Amount Per Serving	
Calories 113	
Total Fat 0g	
Cholesterol 3mg	
Sodium 128mg	
Total Carbohydrate 19g	
Dietary Fiber 0g	
Sugars 18g	
Protein 9g	

Fresh Fruit Smoothie

1½ cups fat-free vanilla yogurt
1 cup fresh blueberries
1 cup fresh peeled peach slices

1. Pulse all ingredients in blender until smooth.

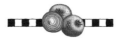

Nutrition Facts	
Serving Size ¾ cup	
Servings Per Recipe 4	
Amount Per Serving	
Calories 76	
Total Fat 0g	
Cholesterol 2mg	
Sodium 38mg	
Total Carbohydrate 17g	
Dietary Fiber 1g	
Sugars 12g	
Protein 3g	

Sugar-free does not mean calorie-free. Be sure to check the nutrition label when buying sugar-free products.

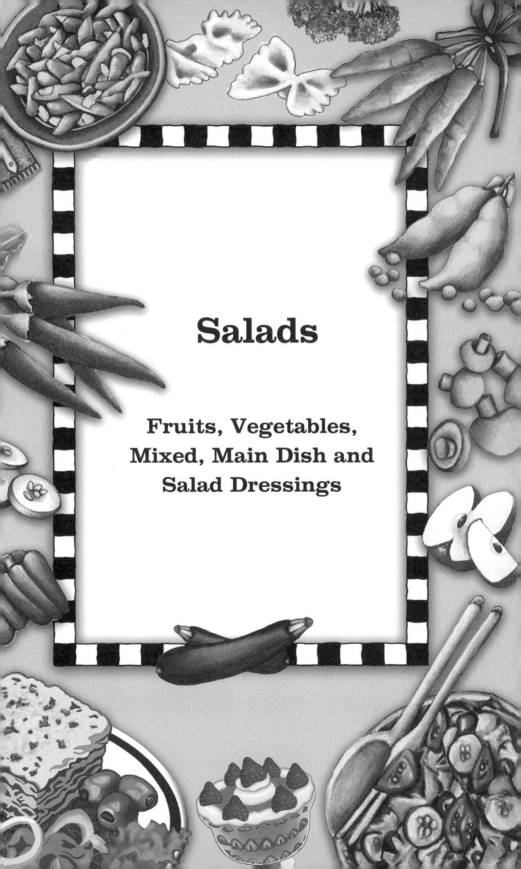

Salads

Fruits, Vegetables, Mixed, Main Dish and Salad Dressings

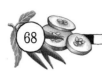

Salads Contents

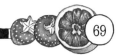

Fruit Medley

1 medium orange
1 large apple with peel, cored, cut into
    ¼-inch wedges
1 banana, peeled, sliced
½ cup fat-free vanilla yogurt

1. Grate 2 teaspoons peel from orange and remove all peel. Separate orange into sections. Arrange fruit on 4 salad plates.

2. Spoon yogurt over fruit and garnish with orange peel.

Nutrition Facts	
Serving Size ½ cup Servings Per Recipe 4	
Amount Per Serving	
Calories 77	
Total Fat 0g	
Cholesterol 0mg	
Sodium 21mg	
Total Carbohydrate 19	
Dietary Fiber 2g	
Sugars 14g	
Protein 2g	

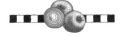

Grapefruit Poppy Seed Salad

4 cups shredded leaf lettuce
1 (20 ounce) jar refrigerated pink grapefruit
    sections, drained
½ cup thinly sliced red onion rings
¼ cup "Poppy Seed Dressing," p. 96

1. Line 4 salad plates with shredded lettuce. Arrange grapefruit and onion on top and drizzle with dressing.

Nutrition Facts	
Serving Size 1 cup Servings Per Recipe 4	
Amount Per Serving	
Calories 119	
Total Fat 6g	
Cholesterol 0mg	
Sodium 14mg	
Total Carbohydrate 16g	
Dietary Fiber 1g	
Sugars14g	
Protein 2g	

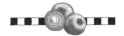

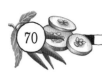

Avocado-Grapefruit Salad

4 cups mixed baby greens
1 Hass avocado, halved, seeded, peeled
1½ cups refrigerated pink grapefruit sections
4 tablespoons fat-free vinaigrette dressing

1. Divide greens among salad plates. Slice
   avocado in thin wedges. Arrange wedges
   and grapefruit sections on greens. Drizzle
   with dressing.

Nutrition Facts	
Serving Size 1½ cups	
Servings Per Recipe 4	
Amount Per Serving	
Calories 138	
Total Fat 7g	
Cholesterol 0mg	
Sodium 507mg	
Total Carbohydrate 17g	
Dietary Fiber 6g	
Sugars 9g	
Protein 3g	

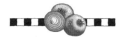

Maybe the little things, like having a meal at the table, are more important than we realize. Maybe these little things are really big things we never forget...big things like memories and family traditions that last a lifetime.

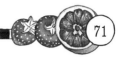
Creamy Cottage Cheese Salad

1 (8 ounce) carton reduced-fat small curd
    cottage cheese
1 (.3 ounce) package instant sugar-free lime
    gelatin mix
1 (8 ounce) container frozen reduced-fat
    whipped topping, thawed
1 (8 ounce) can crushed pineapple, drained

Nutrition Facts	
Serving Size ½ cup	
Servings Per Recipe 8	
Amount Per Serving	
Calories 73	
Total Fat 2g	
Cholesterol 3mg	
Sodium 120mg	
Total Carbohydrate 11g	
Dietary Fiber 0g	
Sugars 7g	
Protein 3g	

1. Spoon cottage cheese in wire mesh strainer
   over medium bowl. Refrigerate 1 hour or
   until well drained.

2. Stir cottage cheese and lime gelatin in large
   bowl. Mix in whipped topping and pineapple.

3. Refrigerate at least 1 hour before serving.

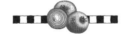

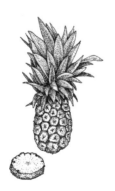

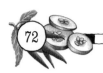

Pineapple-Apple Salad

1 (8 ounce) can crushed pineapple in juice,
    drained
1 (8 ounce) container fat-free frozen whipped
    topping, thawed
1 cup pineapple tidbits, drained
2 cups coarsely chopped apple with peel

1. Mix crushed pineapple and whipped
   topping in large bowl. Stir in pineapple
   tidbits and apple.

Nutrition Facts	
Serving Size ½ cup	
Servings Per Recipe 10	
Amount Per Serving	
Calories 55	
Total Fat 1g	
Cholesterol 0mg	
Sodium 0mg	
Total Carbohydrate 12g	
Dietary Fiber 1g	
Sugars 8g	
Protein 0g	

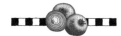

Pistachio-Pineapple Salad

1 (1 ounce) instant sugar-free fat-free pistachio
    pudding mix
1 (8 ounce) can crushed pineapple with juice
1 cup fat-free vanilla yogurt
2½ cups fat-free frozen whipping topping,
    thawed, divided

1. Mix pudding, pineapple and juice and yogurt
   in large bowl until well blended.

2. Stir in 2 cups whipped topping. Cover and
   refrigerate at least 1 hour.

3. Serve ½ cup in small bowls and top with remaining
   whipped topping.

Nutrition Facts	
Serving Size ½ cup	
Servings Per Recipe 8	
Amount Per Serving	
Calories 102	
Total Fat 4g	
Cholesterol 3mg	
Sodium 186mg	
Total Carbohydrate 14g	
Dietary Fiber 0g	
Sugars 11g	
Protein 2g	

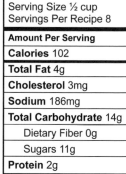

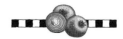

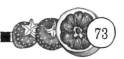

Asparagus and Egg Salad

1 tablespoon canola or olive oil
1 tablespoon fresh lemon juice
1 pound (about 20) fresh asparagus spears,
   trimmed
1 hard-cooked egg white, chopped

Nutrition Facts	
Serving Size 5 spears	
Servings Per Recipe 4	
Amount Per Serving	
Calories 58	
Total Fat 4g	
Cholesterol 0mg	
Sodium 243mg	
Total Carbohydrate 5g	
Dietary Fiber 2g	
Sugars 2g	
Protein 3g	

1. Whisk together oil, lemon juice and
   2 tablespoons water.

2. In 10 to 12-inch skillet over medium-high
   heat, bring ½ cup water to a boil.

3. Add asparagus and cook 3 to 5 minutes, until
   just tender. Remove from heat and cool on paper towels.

4. Arrange asparagus spears on serving platter and drizzle with
   oil-lemon mixture. Garnish with chopped egg.

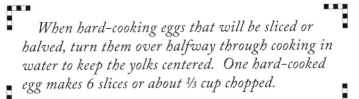

*When hard-cooking eggs that will be sliced or
halved, turn them over halfway through cooking in
water to keep the yolks centered. One hard-cooked
egg makes 6 slices or about ⅓ cup chopped.*

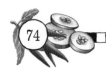

Cauliflower-Tomato Salad

4 cups assorted baby greens
8 cherry tomatoes, halved
1 cup small cauliflower florets
2 tablespoons "Balsamic Vinaigrette," p. 92

1. Mix greens, tomatoes and florets together. Drizzle with dressing and toss lightly.

Nutrition Facts
Serving Size 1 cup
Servings Per Recipe 5
Amount Per Serving
Calories 39
Total Fat 3g
Cholesterol 0mg
Sodium 12mg
Total Carbohydrate 3g
Dietary Fiber 1g
Sugars 1g
Protein 1g

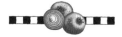

Nature's Favorite Salad

4 large radishes, thinly sliced
1 cup thinly sliced cucumber
½ cup thinly sliced red onion
2 tablespoons "Citrus Vinaigrette
    Dressing," p. 95

1. On 4 salad plates, arrange radishes, cucumber and red onion. Drizzle with dressing.

Nutrition Facts
Serving Size 1 salad
Servings Per Recipe 4
Amount Per Serving
Calories 22
Total Fat 3g
Cholesterol 0mg
Sodium 3mg
Total Carbohydrate 3g
Dietary Fiber 0g
Sugars 1g
Protein 0g

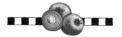

We've all heard the phrase, "cool as a cucumber". Actually, a cucumber's internal temperature is always several degrees cooler than its surroundings.

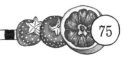

Mediterranean Salad

2 large tomatoes, cut into wedges
⅓ cup red onion slivers
8 large pitted black olives, sliced
2 tablespoons "Feta Cheese Dressing," p. 98

1. Arrange tomatoes, red onion and black olives on 4 salad plates. Drizzle with dressing.

Nutrition Facts
Serving Size ¾ cup
Servings Per Recipe 4
Amount Per Serving
Calories 66
Total Fat 5g
Cholesterol 2mg
Sodium 108mg
Total Carbohydrate 5g
Dietary Fiber 2g
Sugars 3g
Protein 1g

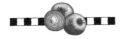

Mediterranean cuisine is the food characteristics of the areas around the Mediterranean Sea. Although there are many regional variations, olives, olive oil, garlic, feta cheese, pita bread and hummus are very popular in the cuisine.

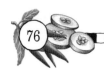

Lucky Black-Eyed Pea Salad

1 (15½ ounce) can black-eyed peas, rinsed,
    drained
⅓ cup finely chopped red onion
½ cup finely chopped red bell pepper
3 tablespoons "Cider Vinaigrette
    Dressing," p. 99

1. Stir together black-eyed peas, onion, pepper
   and dressing in large bowl.

Nutrition Facts	
Serving Size ½ cup	
Servings Per Recipe 5	
Amount Per Serving	
Calories 73	
Total Fat 1g	
Cholesterol 2mg	
Sodium 292mg	
Total Carbohydrate 13g	
Dietary Fiber 3g	
Sugars 1g	
Protein 4g	

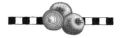

Radish Baby Pea Salad

8 large red lettuce leaves, trimmed
1 cup frozen baby peas, cooked
4 large radishes, sliced
4 tablespoons "Ranch-Style Dressing," p. 97

1. Arrange lettuce leaves, peas and radishes
   on 4 salad plates. Drizzle each salad with
   1 tablespoon dressing.

Nutrition Facts	
Serving Size 1 salad	
Servings Per Recipe 4	
Amount Per Serving	
Calories 70	
Total Fat 3g	
Cholesterol 4mg	
Sodium 254mg	
Total Carbohydrate 9g	
Dietary Fiber 0g	
Sugars 1g	
Protein 1g	

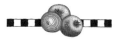

*Generally, the best time to make a radish salad
is in the spring, when radishes are tastiest – mildly
peppery, crisp and juicy.*

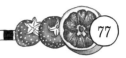
Crunchy Pea Salad

1 (16 ounce) package frozen petite peas
1 cup thinly sliced celery
⅓ cup sliced, rinsed water chestnuts
⅓ cup "Sesame Seed Dressing," p. 77

1. Cook peas according to package directions. Drain and cool.

2. Toss lightly with celery, water chestnuts and dressing.

TIP: Substitute cooked shelled edamame – the Japanese name for green or immature soybeans – which are conveniently available in the freezer section of supermarkets.

Nutrition Facts	
Serving Size ½ cup Servings Per Recipe 8	
Amount Per Serving	
Calories 96	
Total Fat 5g	
Cholesterol 0mg	
Sodium 126mg	
Total Carbohydrate 9g	
Dietary Fiber 3g	
Sugars 4g	
Protein 3g	

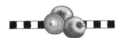

Water chestnuts are a low-sodium choice to add crunch to many recipes. One-half cup water chestnuts canned in water has only 20mg sodium.

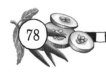

Mushroom Blue Cheese Salad

4 cups torn romaine lettuce leaves
1½ cups sliced fresh white mushrooms
2 tablespoons crumbled blue cheese
2 tablespoons fat-free balsamic vinaigrette
    dressing

1. Line 4 salad plates with lettuce. Top with
    mushrooms and blue cheese and drizzle
    with dressing.

Nutrition Facts	
Serving Size 1½ cups	
Servings Per Recipe 4	
Amount Per Serving	
Calories 30	
Total Fat 1g	
Cholesterol 3mg	
Sodium 104mg	
Total Carbohydrate 3g	
Dietary Fiber 1g	
Sugars 1g	
Protein 2g	

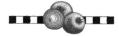

Spinach-Mushroom Crunch Salad

1 (10 ounce) package washed baby spinach
1 cup sliced fresh white mushrooms
2 tablespoons pine nuts, toasted
2 tablespoons fat-free balsamic vinaigrette
    dressing

1. Toss spinach, mushrooms and pine nuts in
    large bowl. Drizzle with dressing, toss lightly
    and serve.

Nutrition Facts	
Serving Size 1 cup	
Servings Per Recipe 6	
Amount Per Serving	
Calories 29	
Total Fat 1g	
Cholesterol 0mg	
Sodium 60mg	
Total Carbohydrate 3g	
Dietary Fiber 1g	
Sugars 0g	
Protein 2g	

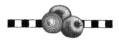

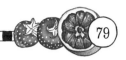
Home-Style Coleslaw

4 cups shredded green cabbage
½ cup slivered green bell pepper
½ cup thinly sliced red onion
¼ cup "Celery Seed Salad Dressing," p. 92

1. Mix cabbage, bell pepper and onion. Drizzle
   with dressing and toss lightly.

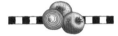

Nutrition Facts
Serving Size ¾ cup
Servings Per Recipe 4
Amount Per Serving
Calories 80
Total Fat 6g
Cholesterol 0mg
Sodium 13mg
Total Carbohydrate 6g
Dietary Fiber 2g
Sugars 3g
Protein 1g

Red Green Crunchy Slaw

2 cups shredded green cabbage
2 cups shredded red cabbage
1 (8 ounce) can sliced water chestnuts,
    rinsed, drained
3 tablespoons "Rice Vinaigrette
    Dressing," p. 95

1. Mix cabbage and water chestnuts in large
   bowl. Drizzle with dressing and toss lightly.

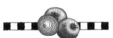

Nutrition Facts
Serving Size ½ cup
Servings Per Recipe 8
Amount Per Serving
Calories 34
Total Fat 1g
Cholesterol 0mg
Sodium 99mg
Total Carbohydrate 6g
Dietary Fiber 2g
Sugars 2g
Protein 1g

*In general, the fewer ingredients in a food
product, the better.*

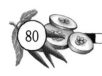

Three Green Slaw

1 (16 ounce) package coleslaw mix
½ cup chopped green bell pepper
¼ cup sliced green onion
⅓ cup "Creamy Slaw Dressing," p. 97

1. Mix coleslaw, pepper and onion in large bowl. Spoon on dressing and toss lightly.

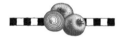

Nutrition Facts
Serving Size 1 cup
Servings Per Recipe 7
Amount Per Serving
Calories 69
Total Fat 2g
Cholesterol 0mg
Sodium 153mg
Total Carbohydrate 11g
Dietary Fiber 4g
Sugars 6g
Protein 3g

The word "coleslaw" is a partial translation from the Dutch term "koosla," which means cabbage slaw. Cabbage salad was a dish known in America by 1785.

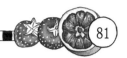
Brown Rice Vegetable Salad

2 cups cooked brown rice
1 cup chopped red bell pepper
½ cup chopped red onion
¼ cup "Feta Cheese Dressing," p. 98

1. Mix all ingredients and refrigerate.

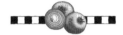

Nutrition Facts	
Serving Size ¾ cup	
Servings Per Recipe 6	
Amount Per Serving	
Calories 102	
Total Fat 2g	
Cholesterol 1mg	
Sodium 14mg	
Total Carbohydrate 18g	
Dietary Fiber 2g	
Sugars 2g	
Protein 2g	

Apple-Walnut Red Cabbage Slaw

1 Granny Smith apple, cored, coarsely chopped
4 cups thinly sliced red cabbage
2 tablespoons chopped walnuts, toasted
¼ cup "Citrus Vinaigrette Dressing," p. 94

1. Toss apple, red cabbage and walnuts. Drizzle with vinaigrette and toss again.

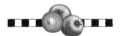

Nutrition Facts	
Serving Size 1 cup	
Servings per Recipe 6	
Amount Per Serving	
Calories 68	
Total Fat 4g	
Cholesterol 0mg	
Sodium 13mg	
Total Carbohydrate 9g	
Dietary Fiber 2g	
Sugars 6g	
Protein 1g	

In 1900, people in the United States chose from 500 or so different foods in grocery stores. More than 50,000 different foods are now available in supermarkets.

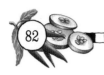

Potluck Apple-Cabbage Mix-Up

1 (16 ounce) package coleslaw mix
2 medium apples with peel, coarsely chopped
¾ cup reduced-fat mayonnaise
3 teaspoons lemon juice

1. Mix slaw and apple in large bowl. Whisk mayonnaise and lemon juice in small bowl and spoon over slaw. Toss lightly.

Nutrition Facts	
Serving Size ¾ cup Servings Per Recipe 12	
Amount Per Serving	
Calories 64	
Total Fat 4g	
Cholesterol 5mg	
Sodium 143mg	
Total Carbohydrate 9g	
Dietary Fiber 2g	
Sugars 5g	
Protein 1g	

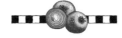

Favorite Waldorf Salad

¼ cup reduced-fat mayonnaise
1 teaspoon lemon juice
2 cups coarsely chopped apple with peel
1 cup thinly sliced celery

1. Whisk mayonnaise and lemon juice in medium bowl. Add apple and celery and toss lightly.

Nutrition Facts	
Serving Size ½ cup Servings Per Recipe 6	
Amount Per Serving	
Calories 48	
Total Fat 2g	
Cholesterol 3mg	
Sodium 101mg	
Total Carbohydrate 7g	
Dietary Fiber 1g	
Sugars 5g	
Protein 0g	

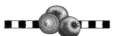

Fat-free does not mean calorie-free.

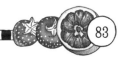

Broccoli-Cranberry Crunchy Slaw

1 (12 ounce) package broccoli slaw, coarsely
    chopped
½ cup dried sweetened cranberries
¼ cup "Best French Dressing," p. 93
¼ cup dry roasted peanuts, coarsely chopped

1. Toss together broccoli slaw, cranberries and
    dressing. Sprinkle peanuts on top.

Nutrition Facts
Serving Size ½ cup
Servings Per Recipe 8
Amount Per Serving
Calories 87
Total Fat 5g
Cholesterol 0mg
Sodium 38mg
Total Carbohydrate 9g
Dietary Fiber 2g
Sugars 6g
Protein 2g

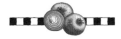

Orange and Red Onion Salad

2 large navel oranges, peeled, sliced
8 thin red onion slices
6 cups torn leaf lettuce
¼ cup fat-free Italian dressing

1. Quarter orange slices and mix with red onion
    and lettuce. Drizzle dressing on top and
    toss lightly.

Nutrition Facts
Serving Size 1 cup
Servings Per Recipe 6
Amount Per Serving
Calories 37
Total Fat 0g
Cholesterol 0mg
Sodium 116mg
Total Carbohydrate 9g
Dietary Fiber 2g
Sugars 6g
Protein 1g

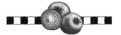

*Substitute 1 teaspoon dried herbs for
1 tablespoon chopped fresh herbs.*

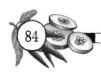

Pear and Feta Green Salad

4 cups mixed baby greens
2 Anjou pears with peel, cored, cut in chunks
   with peel
2 tablespoons crumbled feta cheese
2 tablespoons fat-free balsamic vinaigrette

1. Arrange greens in 4 salad bowls and spoon pears and cheese on top. Drizzle with dressing.

Nutrition Facts	
Serving Size 1 cup	
Servings Per Recipe 4	
Amount Per Serving	
Calories 77	
Total Fat 1g	
Cholesterol 2mg	
Sodium 117mg	
Total Carbohydrate 16g	
Dietary Fiber 4g	
Sugars 10g	
Protein 3g	

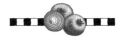

Greek feta cheese has been made for centuries from sheep's or goat's milk. Most feta cheese marketed in the U.S. is made from cow's milk.

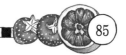

Pineapple-Carrot Slaw

3 medium carrots, peeled, grated
1 cup canned pineapple tidbits in juice, drained
3 cups shredded green cabbage
3 tablespoons fat-free mayonnaise

1. Toss ingredients together in large bowl.
   Cover and refrigerate.

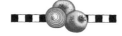

Nutrition Facts	
Serving Size ½ cup	
Servings Per Recipe 6	
Amount Per Serving	
Calories 52	
Total Fat 2g	
Cholesterol 3mg	
Sodium 93mg	
Total Carbohydrate 9g	
Dietary Fiber 2g	
Sugars 6g	
Protein 1g	

Strawberry-Spinach Salad

1 (10 ounce) package washed baby spinach
1½ cups sliced strawberries
2 tablespoons "Balsamic Vinaigrette," p. 92
2 tablespoons chopped pecans, toasted

1. Toss spinach with strawberries in large bowl.
   Drizzle with dressing and sprinkle pecans
   on top.

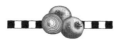

Nutrition Facts	
Serving Size 1 cup	
Servings Per Recipe 5	
Amount Per Serving	
Calories 64	
Total Fat 5g	
Cholesterol 0mg	
Sodium 29mg	
Total Carbohydrate 6g	
Dietary Fiber 2g	
Sugars 3g	
Protein 2g	

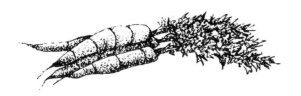

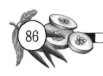

Avocado-Chicken Salad

1 medium avocado
8 cups packaged baby greens
2 cups chopped cooked chicken
4 tablespoons "Balsamic Vinaigrette," p. 92

1. Halve avocado, remove seed, peel and cut in bite-size pieces. Divide greens among 4 plates.

2. Spoon avocado and chicken on greens. Drizzle each salad with 1 tablespoon dressing.

Nutrition Facts	
Serving Size 2½ cups	
Servings Per Recipe 4	
Amount Per Serving	
Calories 243	
Total Fat 12g	
Cholesterol 54mg	
Sodium 98mg	
Total Carbohydrate 8g	
Dietary Fiber 6g	
Sugars 3g	
Protein 24g	

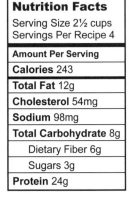

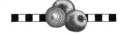

Avocados are a fruit, not a vegetable, as is commonly thought.

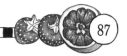

Sesame Chicken Slaw

4 cups shredded green cabbage or coleslaw mix
½ cup finely chopped cooked chicken breast
½ cup sliced water chestnuts, rinsed, drained
3 tablespoons "Sesame Seed Dressing," p. 96

1. Mix cabbage, chicken and water chestnuts
   in large bowl. Drizzle with dressing and
   toss lightly.

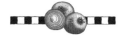

Nutrition Facts	
Serving Size 1½ cups	
Servings Per Recipe 4	
Amount Per Serving	
Calories 85	
Total Fat 4g	
Cholesterol 14mg	
Sodium 90mg	
Total Carbohydrate 7g	
Dietary Fiber 3g	
Sugars 3g	
Protein 6g	

Dilly Chicken Salad

⅓ cup reduced-fat sour cream
1 teaspoon dried dill weed
2 cups shredded cooked chicken breast
½ medium green bell pepper, slivered

1. Stir together sour cream and dill weed. Spoon
   over chicken and bell pepper and mix.

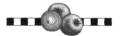

Nutrition Facts	
Serving Size ¾ cup	
Servings Per Recipe 4	
Amount Per Serving	
Calories 125	
Total Fat 2g	
Cholesterol 57mg	
Sodium 70mg	
Total Carbohydrate 3g	
Dietary Fiber 0g	
Sugars 2g	
Protein 22g	

Substitute fresh dill weed whenever possible for dried dill weed. Fresh dill weed has a distinctive, fresher-tasting flavor.

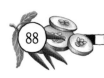

Cranberry-Chicken Salad

2 cups chopped cooked chicken
1 cup chopped celery
⅓ cup dried sweetened cranberries
½ cup reduced-fat mayonnaise

1. Mix all ingredients and refrigerate.

TIP: Substituting fat-free plain yogurt for the reduced-fat mayonnaise reduces calories to 154 and fat to 2 grams per ¾ cup.

Nutrition Facts	
Serving Size ¾ cup	
Servings Per Recipe 4	
Amount Per Serving	
Calories 228	
Total Fat 11g	
Cholesterol 64mg	
Sodium 390mg	
Total Carbohydrate 11g	
Dietary Fiber 1g	
Sugars 7g	
Protein 21g	

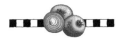

Dried fruits are vitamin-packed but are also concentrated sources of carbohydrate, so keep portions small, such as 2 tablespoons raisins.

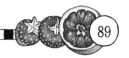
Chicken-Pecan Salad

2 cups finely chopped cooked chicken breast
2 cups thinly sliced celery
¼ cup chopped pecans, toasted
6 tablespoons reduced-fat mayonnaise

1. Mix all ingredients and refrigerate.

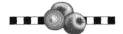

Nutrition Facts	
Serving Size ¾ cup	
Servings Per Recipe 4	
Amount Per Serving	
Calories 213	
Total Fat 12g	
Cholesterol 59mg	
Sodium 280mg	
Total Carbohydrate 4g	
Dietary Fiber 1g	
Sugars 1g	
Protein 21g	

Salad spinners are excellent for removing water from washed greens. Try adding a couple of paper towels to the spinner to speed drying.

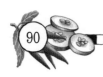

Chicken Caesar Salad

2 (4 ounce) boneless, skinless chicken breast
    halves, grilled or broiled
6 cups torn romaine lettuce
2 tablespoons grated parmesan cheese
2 tablespoons "Amazing Caesar
    Dressing," p. 91

1. Cut cooked chicken breasts in thin strips.
   Divide lettuce among 4 plates and top with
   chicken strips and cheese. Spoon dressing
   on top.

Nutrition Facts	
Serving Size 1 salad	
Servings Per Recipe 4	
Amount Per Serving	
Calories 106	
Total Fat 3g	
Cholesterol 40mg	
Sodium 132mg	
Total Carbohydrate 3g	
Dietary Fiber 1g	
Sugars 1g	
Protein 15g	

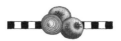

Grape and Turkey Salad

4 cups mixed salad greens
1 cup sliced green or red seedless grapes
2 cups (1-inch cubes) cooked turkey breast
4 tablespoons fat-free raspberry vinaigrette

1. Divide salad greens among 4 salad
   plates. Top each with ¼ cup grapes
   and ½ cup turkey.

2. Drizzle each with 1 tablespoon vinaigrette.

Nutrition Facts	
Serving Size 1 salad	
Servings Per Recipe 4	
Amount Per Serving	
Calories 173	
Total Fat 4g	
Cholesterol 53mg	
Sodium 143mg	
Total Carbohydrate 13g	
Dietary Fiber 2g	
Sugars 11g	
Protein 22g	

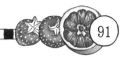

Quick Easy Egg Salad

4 hard-cooked eggs, chopped
½ cup finely chopped celery
⅓ cup reduced-fat mayonnaise
1 teaspoon dijon-style mustard

1. Stir ingredients together. Makes 1¼ cups.

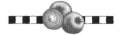

Nutrition Facts	
Serving Size ¼ cup Servings Per Recipe 5	
Amount Per Serving	
Calories 100	
Total Fat 8g	
Cholesterol 174mg	
Sodium 212mg	
Total Carbohydrate 2g	
Dietary Fiber 0g	
Sugars 1g	
Protein 5g	

Amazing Caesar Dressing

⅓ cup fat-free mayonnaise
2 tablespoons lemon juice
2 teaspoons white cooking wine
1 teaspoon dijon-style mustard

1. Stir all ingredients together and refrigerate. Makes ½ cup.

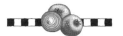

Nutrition Facts	
Serving Size 1 tablespoon Servings Per Recipe 8	
Amount Per Serving	
Calories 24	
Total Fat 2g	
Cholesterol 3mg	
Sodium 104mg	
Total Carbohydrate 1g	
Dietary Fiber 0g	
Sugars 0g	
Protein 0g	

Dijon mustard is made from brown or black mustard seeds, white wine, grape juice and various seasonings. It was originally made in Dijon, France.

Balsamic Vinaigrette

2 tablespoons olive oil
3 tablespoons balsamic vinegar
¼ teaspoon dried basil, crushed
¼ teaspoon dijon-style mustard

1. Whisk all ingredients together. Makes
   ½ cup.

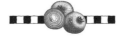

Nutrition Facts	
Serving Size 1 tablespoon	
Servings Per Recipe 8	
Amount Per Serving	
Calories 30	
Total Fat 3g	
Cholesterol 0mg	
Sodium 4mg	
Total Carbohydrate 0g	
Dietary Fiber 0g	
Sugars 0g	
Protein 0g	

Celery Seed Salad Dressing

3 tablespoons canola oil
¼ cup white vinegar
Sugar substitute equal to 2 tablespoons sugar
1 teaspoon celery seed

1. Whisk oil, vinegar and sugar substitute. Stir
   in celery seeds. Makes ½ cup.

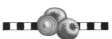

Nutrition Facts	
Serving Size 2 teaspoons	
Servings Per Recipe 10	
Amount Per Serving	
Calories 21	
Total Fat 2g	
Cholesterol 5mg	
Sodium 0mg	
Total Carbohydrate 0g	
Dietary Fiber 0g	
Sugars 0g	
Protein 0g	

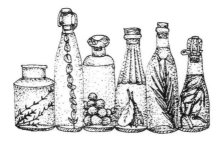

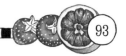
Best French Dressing

½ cup olive oil
¼ cup white or red wine vinegar
1 teaspoon dijon-style mustard
½ teaspoon ground paprika

1. Whisk all ingredients together. Makes
   ¾ cup.

Nutrition Facts		
Serving Size 1 tablespoon		
Servings Per Recipe 12		
Amount Per Serving		
Calories 60		
Total Fat 7g		
Cholesterol 0mg		
Sodium 10mg		
Total Carbohydrate 0g		
Dietary Fiber 0g		
Sugars 0g		
Protein 0g		

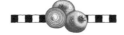

Paprika, the dark reddish powder made by finely grinding sweet red peppers, adds flavor and color to many savory dishes and salad dressings.

Cider Vinaigrette Dressing

2 tablespoons cider vinegar
2 teaspoons canola or olive oil
1 garlic clove, finely minced or pressed
5-10 drops hot pepper sauce

1. Whisk all ingredients together. Makes about 3 tablespoons.

Nutrition Facts		
Serving Size 1 tablespoon		
Servings Per Recipe 3		
Amount Per Serving		
Calories 33		
Total Fat 3g		
Cholesterol 7mg		
Sodium 3mg		
Total Carbohydrate 0g		
Dietary Fiber 0g		
Sugars 0g		
Protein 0g		

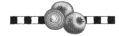

Clean a garlic press right after using it, before any garlic bits left in it dry and clog the holes. A toothbrush is handy for cleaning the clogs.

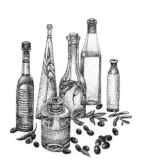

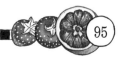

Rice Vinaigrette Dressing

1 tablespoon rice or white wine vinegar
3 tablespoons reduced-sodium soy sauce
1 tablespoon fresh lemon juice
1 tablespoon canola or olive oil

1. Whisk all ingredients together. Makes
   ⅓ cup.

Nutrition Facts	
Serving Size 1 tablespoon	
Servings Per Recipe 5	
Amount Per Serving	
Calories 12	
Total Fat 0g	
Cholesterol 0mg	
Sodium 230mg	
Total Carbohydrate 3g	
Dietary Fiber 0g	
Sugars 1g	
Protein 1g	

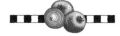

Citrus Vinaigrette Dressing

3 tablespoons fresh orange juice
1 tablespoon fresh lemon juice
2 tablespoons canola or olive oil
Sugar substitute equal to 2 teaspoons sugar

1. Whisk all ingredients together. Makes
   about ⅓ cup.

Nutrition Facts	
Serving Size 1 tablespoon	
Servings Per Recipe 6	
Amount Per Serving	
Calories 43	
Total Fat 5g	
Cholesterol 0mg	
Sodium 0mg	
Total Carbohydrate 1g	
Dietary Fiber 0g	
Sugars 0g	
Protein 0g	

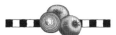

To get more juice from citrus fruit, use the palm of your hand to roll the fruit around on the countertop a few times before cutting and squeezing.

Sesame Seed Dressing

1 tablespoon sesame seeds, toasted
2 tablespoons canola or olive oil
2 tablespoons cider vinegar
1 tablespoon reduced-sodium soy sauce

1. Whisk all ingredients together. Makes about ¼ cup.

Nutrition Facts	
Serving Size 2 teaspoons	
Servings Per Recipe 6	
Amount Per Serving	
Calories 40	
Total Fat 4g	
Cholesterol 0mg	
Sodium 82mg	
Total Carbohydrate 0g	
Dietary Fiber 0g	
Sugars 0g	
Protein 0g	

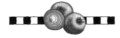

Poppy Seed Dressing

Sugar substitute equal to ⅓ cup sugar
⅓ cup rice or white wine vinegar
¼ cup canola or olive oil
1 tablespoon poppy seeds

1. Whisk together sugar substitute, vinegar, oil and poppy seeds. Makes about ½ cup.

Nutrition Facts	
Serving Size 1 tablespoon	
Servings Per Recipe 8	
Amount Per Serving	
Calories 60	
Total Fat 7g	
Cholesterol 0mg	
Sodium 0mg	
Total Carbohydrate 0g	
Dietary Fiber 0g	
Sugars 0g	
Protein 0g	

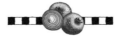

Added sugars in food products are indicated by words ending in "ose," such as fructose, maltose, levulose, and sucrose.

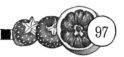

Creamy Slaw Dressing

½ cup reduced-fat mayonnaise
Sugar substitute equal to 1 tablespoon sugar
1 tablespoon cider vinegar
½ teaspoon celery seed

1. Mix ingredients and refrigerate. Makes about ¾ cup.

Nutrition Facts	
Serving Size: 2 teaspoons Servings Per Recipe 12	
Amount Per Serving	
Calories 24	
Total Fat 2g	
Cholesterol 3mg	
Sodium 87mg	
Total Carbohydrate 1g	
Dietary Fiber 0g	
Sugars 0g	
Protein 0g	

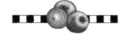

Ranch-Style Dressing

¾ cup reduced-fat mayonnaise
½ cup reduced-fat buttermilk
¼ teaspoon garlic powder
¼ teaspoon onion powder

1. Whisk all ingredients together and refrigerate. Makes about 1 cup.

TIP: To make buttermilk, mix 1 cup milk with 1 tablespoon lemon juice or vinegar and let milk stand for about 10 minutes.

Nutrition Facts	
Serving Size 2 tablespoons Servings Per Recipe 8	
Amount Per Serving	
Calories 62	
Total Fat 5g	
Cholesterol 7mg	
Sodium 219mg	
Total Carbohydrate 3g	
Dietary Fiber 0g	
Sugars 1g	
Protein 1g	

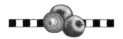

Feta Cheese Dressing

2 tablespoons olive oil
3 tablespoons red wine vinegar
1 teaspoon dried basil, crushed
2 tablespoons crumbled feta cheese

1. Whisk all ingredients together. Makes about ⅓ cup.

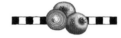

Nutrition Facts	
Serving Size 2 teaspoons	
Servings Per Recipe 6	
Amount Per Serving	
Calories 48	
Total Fat 5g	
Cholesterol 3mg	
Sodium 35mg	
Total Carbohydrate 0g	
Dietary Fiber 0g	
Sugars 0g	
Protein 0g	

Organic versus non-organic: Not all organic foods offer better health values than non-organic, and on average you'll pay 50 percent more for organic foods. However, it is worth paying the price to reduce your exposure to pesticides and other additives for certain foods. As a result of extensive testing, the U.S.D.A. recommends buying organic foods such as apples, nectarines, bell peppers, celery, cucumbers and lettuce or buying from local farmers' markets.

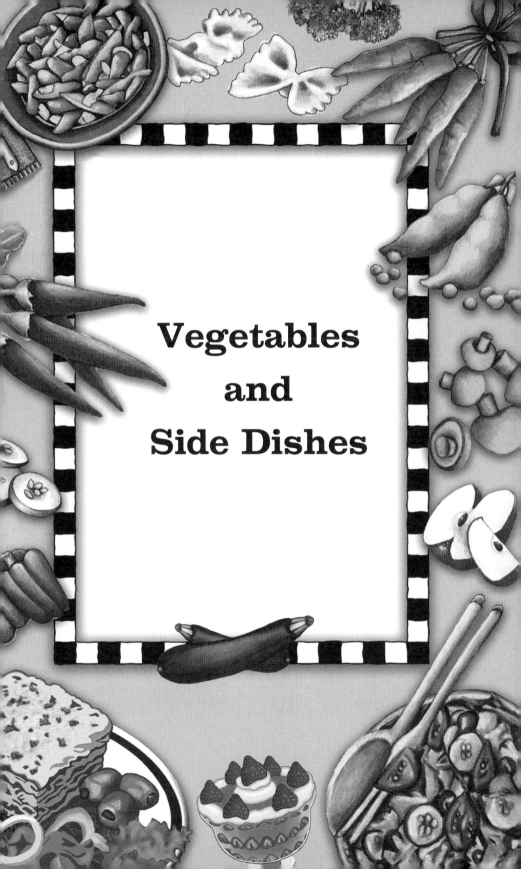

Vegetables
and
Side Dishes

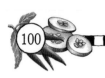

Vegetables and Side Dishes Contents

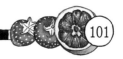
Buttered Spaghetti Squash

1 (3 pound) spaghetti squash
3 tablespoons melted butter

1. Halve squash lengthwise. Remove seeds and loose strings with a spoon or melon baller.

2. Place squash halves in large, heavy pan and cover with water.

3. Bring to a boil, reduce heat and slowly boil squash until tender, about 12 to 15 minutes.

4. Remove squash and drain. When cool enough to handle, pull out strands with fork. Transfer to serving dish and drizzle with melted butter.

Nutrition Facts	
Serving Size ¾ cup	
Servings Per Recipe 6	
Amount Per Serving	
Calories 123	
Total Fat 6g	
Cholesterol 16mg	
Sodium 41mg	
Total Carbohydrate 16g	
Dietary Fiber 0g	
Sugars 0g	
Protein 0g	

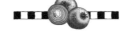

Carrots, squash and sweet potatoes contain beta-carotene, which your body converts to vitamin A. It's vital for proper eyesight and healthy hair and skin.

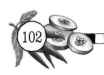
Chinese Cabbage Stir-Fry

1 (2 pound) head Chinese (napa) cabbage
2 cloves garlic, minced
1 tablespoon packed brown sugar
2 teaspoons "Simple Stir-Fry Sauce," p. 218

Nutrition Facts	
Serving Size 1 cup	
Servings Per Recipe 3	
Amount Per Serving	
Calories 54	
Total Fat 1g	
Cholesterol 0mg	
Sodium 70mg	
Total Carbohydrate 11g	
Dietary Fiber 3g	
Sugars 7g	
Protein 3g	

1. Wash, core and quarter cabbage. Thinly slice quarters.

2. Preheat sprayed nonstick wok or nonstick 12-inch skillet on medium-high heat.

3. Add garlic and cook and stir only a few seconds. Add cabbage slices and cook and stir about 3 minutes or until cabbage is tender. Stir in brown sugar and sauce.

You'll find these recipes use a lot of freshly minced garlic that is cooked briefly. This helps reduce the strong, pungent taste of raw garlic.

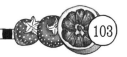

Eggplant and Zucchini

2 cloves garlic, minced
1 cup chopped yellow or red bell pepper
3 cups (1 medium) peeled, (1-inch) cubed
    eggplant
2 medium zucchini, cut in 1-inch pieces

Nutrition Facts		
Serving Size ½ cup		
Servings Per Recipe 8		
Amount Per Serving		
Calories 23		
Total Fat 0g		
Cholesterol 0mg		
Sodium 5mg		
Total Carbohydrate 5g		
Dietary Fiber 2g		
Sugars 3g		
Protein 1g		

1. Cook and stir garlic and bell pepper in sprayed nonstick 10 to 12-inch skillet over medium heat until tender.

2. Add eggplant, zucchini and ½ cup water. Bring to a boil, reduce heat and simmer 10 to 15 minutes or until vegetables become tender.

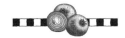

Deodorize a garlicky cutting board by rubbing it with a paste of baking soda and water.

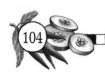

Eggplant Parmesan

1 medium eggplant (1¼ pounds)
½ cup panko (Japanese-style) breadcrumbs
3 tablespoons grated parmesan cheese
2 egg whites, beaten

Nutrition Facts		
Serving Size 2 slices Servings Per Recipe 6		
Amount Per Serving		
Calories 44		
Total Fat 1g		
Cholesterol 2mg		
Sodium 81mg		
Total Carbohydrate 5g		
Dietary Fiber 3g		
Sugars 2g		
Protein 4g		

1. Slice eggplant into ⅜-inch slices with peel on. Sprinkle with 1 tablespoon salt and let drain into colander for 30 minutes. Rinse well and pat dry.

2. Preheat oven to 375°.

3. Combine breadcrumbs and cheese. Dip eggplant slices in egg and coat with crumbs.

4. Place on sprayed foil-lined baking sheet. Bake 20 to 25 minutes or until eggplant becomes tender.

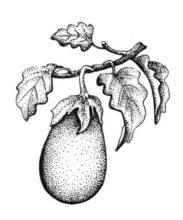

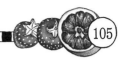

Gingered Broccoli

4 cups small broccoli florets
6 thin slices peeled fresh ginger root
1 clove garlic, minced
1 tablespoon reduced-sodium soy sauce

1. In electric steamer or in large, heavy pan with steamer basket, steam broccoli until just tender.

2. In sprayed nonstick 10 to 12-inch skillet over medium heat, cook and stir ginger and garlic about 1 minute.

3. Add soy sauce and heat about 2 minutes. Remove ginger and spoon sauce over broccoli.

Nutrition Facts	
Serving Size 1 cup	
Servings Per Recipe 4	
Amount Per Serving	
Calories 37	
Total Fat 0g	
Cholesterol 0mg	
Sodium 175mg	
Total Carbohydrate 7g	
Dietary Fiber 2g	
Sugars 2g	
Protein 3g	

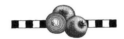

Fresh ginger math – a 2-inch piece of peeled ginger will make 2 tablespoons minced.

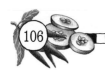

Golden Top-Broiled Tomatoes

4 medium firm, ripe tomatoes
½ cup reduced-fat mayonnaise
1 tablespoon grated parmesan cheese
4 green onion tops, finely chopped

Nutrition Facts	
Serving Size 1 tomato half Servings Per Recipe 8	
Amount Per Serving	
Calories 49	
Total Fat 4g	
Cholesterol 4mg	
Sodium 144mg	
Total Carbohydrate 4g	
Dietary Fiber 1g	
Sugars 2g	
Protein 1g	

1. Core tomatoes and slice in half horizontally. Arrange on sprayed foil-lined baking sheet. Preheat broiler.

2. Mix mayonnaise, cheese and onion. Spread 1 tablespoon on each tomato half.

3. Place tomato halves on sprayed foil-lined baking sheet. Broil about 5 inches from heat until topping puffs and is golden.

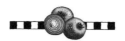

Green Beans Dijon

1 (16 ounce) package frozen cut green beans
3 teaspoons lemon juice
1 teaspoon dijon-style mustard
1 tablespoon toasted chopped walnuts

Nutrition Facts	
Serving Size ½ cup Servings Per Recipe 4	
Amount Per Serving	
Calories 57	
Total Fat 1g	
Cholesterol 0mg	
Sodium 30mg	
Total Carbohydrate 8g	
Dietary Fiber 0g	
Sugars 0g	
Protein 0g	

1. Cook green beans according to package instructions. Stir lemon juice and mustard together and toss with green beans. Sprinkle with walnuts.

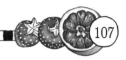
Grilled Eggplant

1 medium eggplant (1¼ pounds)
½ cup "Balsamic Vinaigrette," p. 92

1. Peel and slice eggplant into ⅜ inch slices.
   Sprinkle with 1 tablespoon salt and let drain
   into colander for 30 minutes. Rinse well and
   pat dry.

2. Transfer eggplant to shallow baking dish and
   spoon dressing on top. Marinate 15 minutes
   and turn once. Drain.

3. Grill eggplant on gas or charcoal grill, turning
   occasionally, until tender, about 10 to 15 minutes.

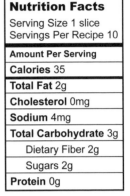

Nutrition Facts	
Serving Size 1 slice	
Servings Per Recipe 10	
Amount Per Serving	
Calories 35	
Total Fat 2g	
Cholesterol 0mg	
Sodium 4mg	
Total Carbohydrate 3g	
Dietary Fiber 2g	
Sugars 2g	
Protein 0g	

"Good" carbs come from fruits, vegetables
and whole grains. They keep your cholesterol
level healthy and your blood pressure and blood
sugar stable.

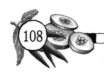

Italian Green Beans

2 cups frozen cut green beans
1 cup finely chopped onion
2 garlic cloves, minced
1 (15 ounce) can Italian stewed tomatoes

Nutrition Facts	
Serving Size ½ cup	
Servings Per Recipe 4	
Amount Per Serving	
Calories 71	
Total Fat 0g	
Cholesterol 0mg	
Sodium 317mg	
Total Carbohydrate 14g	
Dietary Fiber 4g	
Sugars 8g	
Protein 2g	

1. Cook green beans according to package instructions.

2. In sprayed nonstick 10 to 12-inch skillet on medium heat, cook and stir onion and garlic until tender.

3. Pour in tomatoes and bring to a boil. Reduce heat and simmer, covered, about 10 to 12 minutes.

4. Stir in beans and heat through.

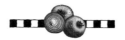

When cooking garlic and onions, cook the onions until almost done, then add the garlic and cook briefly.

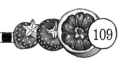
Lemon-Butter Baby Green Beans

1 (14 ounce) package frozen whole baby green beans
1 tablespoon butter
¼ cup slivered almonds
1 tablespoon lemon juice

Nutrition Facts		
Serving Size ½ cup		
Servings Per Recipe 6		
Amount Per Serving		
Calories 69		
Total Fat 4g		
Cholesterol 5mg		
Sodium 32mg		
Total Carbohydrate 5g		
Dietary Fiber 2g		
Sugars 2g		
Protein 2g		

1. Cook green beans according to package instructions. Drain and transfer to serving dish.

2. In 6 to 8-inch skillet on medium heat, cook and stir butter and almonds until almonds brown. (Be careful not to burn.)

3. Stir in lemon juice and pour over green beans.

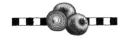

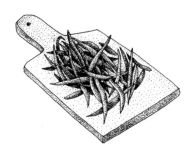

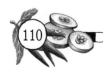

Lemon-Thyme Roasted Asparagus

2 pounds (about 30 spears) fresh asparagus,
    trimmed
2 teaspoons olive oil
½ teaspoon dried thyme, crushed
½ teaspoon grated lemon peel

Nutrition Facts	
Serving size 1 cup	
Servings Per Recipe 6	
Amount Per Serving	
Calories 44	
Total Fat 2g	
Cholesterol 0mg	
Sodium 3mg	
Total Carbohydrate 6g	
Dietary Fiber 3g	
Sugars 3g	
Protein 3g	

1. Preheat oven to 450°.

2. Spread asparagus spears on foil-lined baking sheet. Sprinkle with oil, thyme and lemon peel and toss to coat.

3. Bake for 10 minutes, stirring once, until just tender.

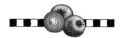

> *Fresh herbs, when available, are preferable to dried herbs. When you use dried herbs, measure the amount needed and crush between your fingers to release stored-up flavors.*

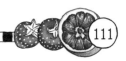

Mashed Sweet Potatoes

2 large sweet potatoes
2 teaspoons ground cinnamon
1 tablespoon grated orange peel
2 tablespoons sugar-free maple syrup

1. Scrub sweet potatoes and prick skins. Cover and cook in microwave on HIGH for 4 minutes on each side or until potatoes are soft. Let stand 1 to 2 minutes.

2. Scoop potato from shells and mash with fork. Stir in cinnamon, orange peel and maple syrup.

Nutrition Facts
Serving Size ½ cup
Servings Per Recipe 4
Amount Per Serving
Calories 66
Total Fat 0g
Cholesterol 0mg
Sodium 50mg
Total Carbohydrate 16g
Dietary Fiber 3g
Sugars 3g
Protein 1g

Contrary to popular belief, sweet potatoes are not related to yams. Some confusion began in the 1930's when Louisiana hit on "yams" to distinguish their sweet potatoes from the drier, paler sweet potatoes grown in New Jersey, Maryland and Virginia.

Mediterranean Vegetable Mix

3 cups (1 medium) peeled, cubed eggplant
   (1-inch cubes)
2 cups sliced zucchini
2 cups sliced small white mushrooms
1 (15 ounce) can diced tomatoes with basil,
   oregano and garlic

1. In sprayed nonstick 10 to 12-inch skillet
   over medium heat, cook and stir eggplant,
   zucchini and mushrooms about 5 minutes.

2. Add tomatoes to skillet and bring to a boil.
   Reduce heat and simmer about 20 minutes
   or until vegetables become tender.

Nutrition Facts	
Serving Size ½ cup	
Servings Per Recipe 8	
Amount Per Serving	
Calories 38	
Total Fat 0g	
Cholesterol 0mg	
Sodium 28mg	
Total Carbohydrate 16g	
Dietary Fiber 7g	
Sugars 9g	
Protein 3g	

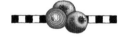

Okra and Tomatoes

1 cup chopped onion
½ cup chopped green bell pepper
1 (16 ounce) package sliced frozen okra,
   cooked, drained
2 (15 ounce) cans diced tomatoes with garlic,
   oregano and basil

1. In sprayed nonstick 10 to 12-inch skillet on
   medium heat, cook and stir onion and bell
   pepper about 4 to 5 minutes or until tender.

2. Add okra and tomatoes and heat through.

Nutrition Facts	
Serving Size ½ cup	
Servings Per Recipe 8	
Amount Per Serving	
Calories 49	
Total Fat 0g	
Cholesterol 0mg	
Sodium 25mg	
Total Carbohydrate 10g	
Dietary Fiber 2g	
Sugars 6g	
Protein 2g	

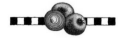

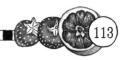
Cheesy Microwave Cauliflower

1 (2 pound) cauliflower
¾ cup shredded reduced-fat cheddar cheese
Paprika for garnish

Nutrition Facts		
Serving Size ½ cup		
Servings Per Recipe 6		
Amount Per Serving		
Calories 60		
Total Fat 1g		
Cholesterol 3mg		
Sodium 129mg		
Total Carbohydrate 7g		
Dietary Fiber 3g		
Sugars 3g		
Protein 6g		

1. Trim leaves, cut off stem and leave cauliflower whole.

2. In microwave-safe 1½ to 2-quart dish, add 2 tablespoons water and cauliflower.

3. Cover and microwave on HIGH for about 9 minutes, turning dish once. Cauliflower should be just tender.

4. Drain cauliflower, sprinkle with cheese and let stand until cheese melts. Sprinkle with paprika.

TIP: *Since cauliflower tends to be expensive, look for clean, white clusters and green leaves. One medium head, about 2 pounds, makes 4 to 6 generous portions.*

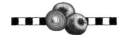

For best flavor and fewer seeds, choose small zucchini – about 4 to 6-inches long. Look for smooth, unblemished skin. One pound zucchini will yield 4 cups of sliced zucchini.

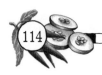

Roasted Mixed Vegetables

2 medium zucchini, quartered lengthwise
1 (1 pound) eggplant, peeled, cut in
    ½-inch slices
1 medium red onion, cut in ½-inch slices
½ cup crumbled feta cheese

1. Preheat oven to 400°.

2. Spread vegetables on sprayed foil-lined baking sheet.

3. Bake vegetables for 20 to 25 minutes; stir once. Cut into bite-size pieces and sprinkle with cheese.

Nutrition Facts	
Serving Size ½ cup	
Servings Per Recipe 8	
Amount Per Serving	
Calories 50	
Total Fat 1g	
Cholesterol 4mg	
Sodium 111mg	
Total Carbohydrate 6g	
Dietary Fiber 3g	
Sugars 3g	
Protein 3g	

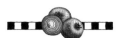

Blue or gorgonzola cheeses are good substitutes for the rich, tangy flavor of feta cheese.

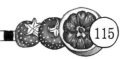

Simple Stir-Fry Snow Peas

1 (8 ounce) package fresh snow peas
1 teaspoon olive oil
2 cloves garlic, minced
2 teaspoons reduced-sodium soy sauce

1. Rinse and remove ends and strings from snow peas.

2. Heat oil in 6 to 8-inch skillet on medium-high heat and cook and stir garlic just a few seconds.

3. Add snow peas and soy sauce and cook about 1 to 2 minutes.

Nutrition Facts	
Serving Size ½ cup	
Servings Per Recipe 3	
Amount Per Serving	
Calories 48	
Total Fat 2g	
Cholesterol 0mg	
Sodium 129mg	
Total Carbohydrate 6g	
Dietary Fiber 2g	
Sugars 3g	
Protein 2g	

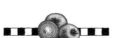

Clean a garlic press right after using it, before any garlic bits left in it dry and clog the holes. A toothbrush is handy for cleaning the clogs.

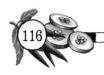

Snap Pea and Carrot Stir-Fry

2 garlic cloves, minced
2 cups diagonally sliced carrots
1 (16 ounce) package frozen sugar snap peas,
    slightly thawed
1 tablespoon reduced-sodium soy sauce

Nutrition Facts
Serving Size ½ cup
Servings Per Recipe 4
Amount Per Serving
Calories 74
Total Fat 0g
Cholesterol 0mg
Sodium 199mg
Total Carbohydrate 14g
Dietary Fiber 4g
Sugars 8g
Protein 3g

1. In sprayed nonstick wok or 10 to 12-inch skillet over medium-high heat, cook and stir garlic and carrots for 3 to 4 minutes.

2. Increase heat to medium-high and add sugar snap peas.

3. Add soy sauce, cook and stir until carrots and peas are just tender.

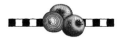

Garlic math – 1 medium clove makes ½ teaspoon minced.

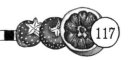

Snow Peas and Red Bell Pepper

2 cloves garlic, minced
1 large red bell pepper, slivered
1 (8 ounce) package fresh snow peas, strings
    removed
2 teaspoons sesame seeds, toasted

Nutrition Facts		
Serving Size ½ cup Servings Per Recipe 4		
Amount Per Serving		
Calories 46		
Total Fat 1g		
Cholesterol 0mg		
Sodium 2mg		
Total Carbohydrate 7g		
Dietary Fiber 2g		
Sugars 4g		
Protein 2g		

1. In sprayed nonstick 10 to 12-inch skillet over medium heat, cook and stir garlic and bell pepper until tender.

2. Add snow peas and cook and stir for about 2 minutes. Transfer to serving dish and sprinkle with sesame seeds.

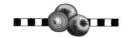

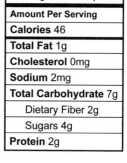

> *Weight Management: Eat small portions. If you eat a restaurant meal, take home half for lunch tomorrow.*

Stuffed Mushrooms

12 large white mushrooms
1 tablespoon reduced-fat cream cheese
½ teaspoon Italian herb seasoning, crushed
2 tablespoons toasted "Lite Wheat
    Breadcrumbs," p. 226

Nutrition Facts		
Serving Size 2 mushrooms		
Servings Per Recipe 6		
Amount Per Serving		
Calories 19		
Total Fat 1g		
Cholesterol 2mg		
Sodium 26mg		
Total Carbohydrate 3g		
Dietary Fiber 1g		
Sugars 1g		
Protein 2g		

1. Preheat oven to 350°.

2. Remove stems from mushroom caps
   and chop finely. Place caps on sprayed
   foil-lined baking pan.

3. In sprayed nonstick 6 to 8-inch skillet over
   medium heat, cook and stir chopped mushroom stems
   for 2 to 3 minutes.

4. Stir in cream cheese, herbs and breadcrumbs. Cook and stir for
   1 to 2 minutes.

5. Spoon mushroom stem mixture evenly into mushroom caps
   and spray.

6. Cover baking pan with foil and bake about 15 minutes or until
   caps are tender. Remove foil and bake 5 to 6 minutes or until
   tops brown.

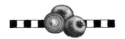

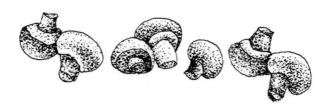

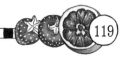
Yellow Squash Casserole

2 pounds yellow crookneck squash, thinly sliced
¾ cup shredded reduced-fat cheddar cheese, divided
¼ cup reduced-fat mayonnaise
¼ cup liquid egg substitute

Nutrition Facts
Serving Size ½ cup
Servings Per Recipe 9
Amount Per Serving
Calories 54
Total Fat 2g
Cholesterol 4mg
Sodium 131mg
Total Carbohydrate 5g
Dietary Fiber 1g
Sugars 4g
Protein 4g

1. Cover squash with water and bring to a boil in 2 to 3-quart saucepan.

2. Cook 8 to 10 minutes or until just tender. Drain well in strainer and press out liquid with fingers.

3. Preheat oven to 350°.

4. Combine drained squash, ½ cup cheese, mayonnaise and egg substitute. Spoon into sprayed 1½ to 2-quart baking dish.

5. Sprinkle with remaining ¼ cup cheese and bake uncovered about 30 minutes.

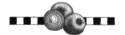

Carrots, squash and sweet potatoes contain beta-carotene, which your body converts to vitamin A. It's vital for proper eyesight and healthy hair and skin.

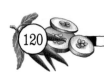

Zucchini with Cherry Tomatoes

4 medium zucchini, sliced
1 tablespoon butter
1 cup halved cherry tomatoes
½ teaspoon dried basil

Nutrition Facts		
Serving Size ½ cup		
Servings Per Recipe 6		
Amount Per Serving		
Calories 35		
Total Fat 2g		
Cholesterol 5mg		
Sodium 8mg		
Total Carbohydrate 3g		
Dietary Fiber 1g		
Sugars 3g		
Protein 1g		

1. To sprayed nonstick 10 to 12-inch skillet, add zucchini and 1 cup water. Bring to a boil and reduce heat.

2. Simmer, covered, until zucchini is just tender, about 4 minutes.

3. Remove zucchini and water from skillet and drain zucchini.

4. Melt butter in same skillet over medium heat. Add zucchini, tomatoes and basil and simmer about 1 minute or until tomatoes are hot.

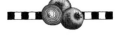

Basil was called the royal herb by ancient Greeks. It gives Mediterranean dishes a characteristic flavor and is an essential ingredient in pesto.

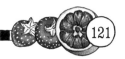

Asparagus with Bacon

1 pound asparagus, trimmed
2 tablespoons fat-free vinaigrette dressing
4 slices turkey bacon, cooked, crumbled

1. Place asparagus in 10 to 12-inch skillet and add enough water to cover asparagus.

2. Bring to a boil, reduce heat and cook until just tender. Remove and drain.

3. Sprinkle asparagus with dressing and lightly toss. Cover and refrigerate about 30 minutes.

4. Divide into 4 servings and sprinkle with bacon crumbles.

Nutrition Facts
Serving Size 1 cup (about 5 spears)
Servings Per Recipe 4
Amount Per Serving
Calories 59
Total Fat 3g
Cholesterol 10mg
Sodium 462mg
Total Carbohydrate 5g
Dietary Fiber 2g
Sugars 2g
Protein 4g

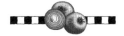

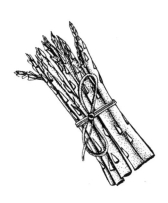

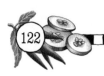

Asparagus with Toasted Almonds

1¼ pounds fresh asparagus, trimmed
2 tablespoons lemon juice
1 tablespoon slivered almonds, toasted

Nutrition Facts	
Serving Size 1 cup	
Servings Per Recipe 4	
Amount Per Serving	
Calories 40	
Total Fat 1g	
Cholesterol 0mg	
Sodium 287mg	
Total Carbohydrate 7g	
Dietary Fiber 3g	
Sugars 3g	
Protein 4g	

1. Add asparagus and enough water to cover asparagus in 10 to 12-inch skillet and bring to a boil.

2. Reduce heat to simmer and cook, uncovered, about 5 to 7 minutes or until asparagus is just tender.

3. Drain and transfer to serving dish. Sprinkle with lemon juice and garnish with almonds.

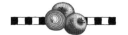

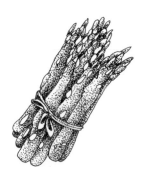

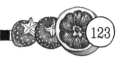
Baked Balsamic Onions

2 large white or yellow onions, cut into
   1-inch wedges
3 tablespoons fat-free balsamic vinaigrette
1 teaspoon dried thyme, crushed
1 tablespoon grated parmesan cheese

Nutrition Facts
Serving Size ½ cup
Servings Per Recipe 6
Amount Per Serving
Calories 31
Total Fat 0g
Cholesterol 1mg
Sodium 17mg
Total Carbohydrate 6g
Dietary Fiber 1g
Sugars 3g
Protein 1g

1. Preheat oven to 425°.

2. Arrange onion wedges to overlap slightly in sprayed 9 x 13-inch baking dish.

3. Drizzle vinaigrette over onions and sprinkle with thyme.

4. Bake, uncovered, about 45 minutes or until onions become tender. Sprinkle with cheese.

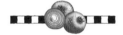

Home gives us a sense of place and a sense of who we are.

Baked Parmesan Tomatoes

2 slices light-style wheat bread
4 medium tomatoes, halved
3 tablespoons grated parmesan cheese
1 teaspoon dried basil, crushed

Nutrition Facts	
Serving Size 1 tomato half	
Servings Per Recipe 8	
Amount Per Serving	
Calories 34	
Total Fat 1g	
Cholesterol 2mg	
Sodium 67mg	
Total Carbohydrate 4g	
Dietary Fiber 1g	
Sugars 2g	
Protein 3g	

1. Preheat oven to 375°.

2. Process bread in blender, one slice at a time, to make soft breadcrumbs.

3. Arrange tomato halves in shallow baking pan. Mix breadcrumbs, cheese and basil and sprinkle over tomato halves.

4. Bake 15 to 20 minutes or until topping browns.

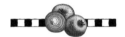

When a recipe calls for parmesan cheese, freshly grated parmesan cheese is preferred over the dry, powdery parmesan cheese in shaker cans.

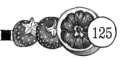
Balsamic Brussels Sprouts

1 (2 pint) carton fresh Brussels sprouts,
    trimmed
1 tablespoon olive oil
1 medium onion, thinly sliced
¼ cup balsamic vinegar

Nutrition Facts	
Serving Size ½ cup	
Servings Per Recipe 4	
Amount Per Serving	
Calories 79	
Total Fat 4g	
Cholesterol 0mg	
Sodium 23mg	
Total Carbohydrate 10g	
Dietary Fiber 4g	
Sugars 3g	
Protein 3g	

1. In 3 to 4-quart saucepan, bring 2 quarts water to a boil. Add sprouts and reduce heat to medium.

2. Cook for 20 minutes or until sprouts are fork-tender; drain.

3. In 10 to 12-inch skillet on medium heat, cook and stir olive oil and onion until onion is tender.

4. Add vinegar and drained sprouts. Stir to coat sprouts and heat through.

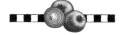

Traditionally, balsamic vinegar is made in Italy from white grapes which are cooked and concentrated, until deep, dark and rich. The flavor and color are deepened further by a long aging process in wooden barrels.

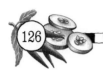

Bok Choy-Onion Stir-Fry

1 (1 pound) head bok choy
1 medium onion, thinly sliced
1 teaspoon packed brown sugar
2 teaspoons "Simple Stir-Fry Sauce," p. 218

Nutrition Facts
Serving Size 1 cup
Servings Per Recipe 4
Amount Per Serving
Calories 33
Total Fat 1g
Cholesterol 0mg
Sodium 123mg
Total Carbohydrate 6g
Dietary Fiber 2g
Sugars 4g
Protein 2g

1. Separate bok choy leaves, wash thoroughly and cut stalks away from leaves.

2. Cut stalks into ½-inch diagonal pieces. Roll leaves and shred ¼-inch wide.

3. Add bok choy stalk pieces and onion to sprayed nonstick 10 to 12-inch skillet over medium-high heat. Cook and stir about 5 minutes.

4. Add leaves, brown sugar and 2 tablespoons water. Cover and steam about 2 minutes or until leaves wilt. Uncover and toss with sauce.

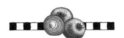

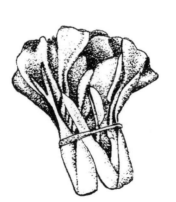

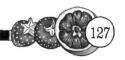
Broccoli-Mushroom Stir-Fry

1 pound fresh small broccoli florets
1 cup sliced small white mushrooms
2 green onions, sliced
¼ cup toasted slivered almonds

Nutrition Facts		
Serving Size ¾ cup		
Servings Per Recipe 6		
Amount Per Serving		
Calories 55		
Total Fat 3g		
Cholesterol 0mg		
Sodium 26mg		
Total Carbohydrate 7g		
Dietary Fiber 3g		
Sugars 2g		
Protein 3g		

1. Preheat sprayed nonstick 10 to 12-inch skillet on medium-high heat. When hot, add broccoli and stir-fry 1 minute.

2. Add 1 tablespoon water, cover and cook about 3 minutes or until broccoli becomes tender. Remove broccoli from skillet.

3. In same skillet on medium heat, cook and stir mushrooms and green onions about 3 minutes.

4. Return broccoli to skillet and heat through. Sprinkle with almonds.

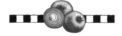

When a recipe calls for mushrooms, choose fresh, small to medium white mushrooms. However, fresh small portobello mushrooms may be substituted for white mushrooms in most recipes.

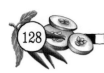

Browned Brussels Sprouts

1 (2-pint) carton Brussels sprouts, trimmed
2 garlic cloves, minced
2 teaspoons olive oil
1 tablespoon lemon juice

Nutrition Facts	
Serving Size 6 sprout halves	
Servings Per Recipe 4	
Amount Per Serving	
Calories 61	
Total Fat 3g	
Cholesterol 0mg	
Sodium 22mg	
Total Carbohydrate 9g	
Dietary Fiber 3g	
Sugars 2g	
Protein 3g	

1. Bring 2 quarts water to a boil in 3 to 4-quart saucepan.

2. Add sprouts, reduce heat to medium and cook for 20 minutes or until sprouts become tender. Drain sprouts and cut in quarters.

3. Add olive oil, garlic and sprouts to nonstick 10 to 12-inch skillet on medium heat.

4. Cook, stirring occasionally, until sprouts become brown in spots. Remove from heat and sprinkle with lemon juice.

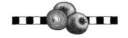

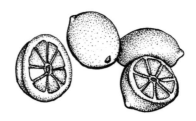

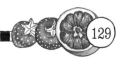

Yellow Rice and Broccoli

1 (5 ounce) package saffron yellow rice
2 cups small broccoli florets
¼ cup diced pimiento, drained
1 tablespoon finely chopped fresh parsley

1. Follow package directions to prepare yellow rice. Steam broccoli in electric steamer or in steamer basket in large, heavy pan.

2. In large, heavy pan over medium heat, stir rice, broccoli, pimiento and parsley. Heat through.

Nutrition Facts	
Serving Size ½ cup	
Servings Per Recipe 10	
Amount Per Serving	
Calories 56	
Total Fat 0g	
Cholesterol 0mg	
Sodium 194mg	
Total Carbohydrate 12g	
Dietary Fiber 1g	
Sugars 1g	
Protein 2g	

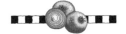

Broccoli is a super hero of nutrition! A ½-cup serving of cooked broccoli provides plenty of vitamins A and C, folic acid, calcium and iron – for only 22 calories.

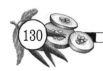

Vegetarian Green Chile Rice

2¼ cups reduced-sodium vegetable broth
1 cup brown rice
1 (4 ounce) can diced green chilies
½ cup shredded reduced-fat cheddar cheese

1. Bring broth to boiling in 3 to 4-quart saucepan. Stir in rice and reduce heat to simmer about 1 hour or until rice is tender.

2. Stir in chilies and cheese. Remove heat, cover and let stand about 5 minutes.

Nutrition Facts	
Serving Size ½ cup Servings Per Recipe 8	
Amount Per Serving	
Calories 107	
Total Fat 1g	
Cholesterol 0mg	
Sodium 236mg	
Total Carbohydrate 20g	
Dietary Fiber 1g	
Sugars 1g	
Protein 4g	

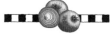

Spanish Brown Rice

1 cup chopped onion
1 cup chopped bell pepper
1 (8 ounce) can tomato sauce with
    roasted garlic
2 cups cooked brown rice

1. In sprayed nonstick 10 to 12-inch skillet over medium-high heat, cook and stir onion and bell pepper until tender.

2. Stir in tomato sauce and brown rice and heat through.

Nutrition Facts	
Serving Size ½ cup Servings Per Recipe 8	
Amount Per Serving	
Calories 73	
Total Fat 0g	
Cholesterol 0mg	
Sodium 172mg	
Total Carbohydrate 16g	
Dietary Fiber 2g	
Sugars 2g	
Protein 2g	

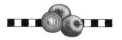

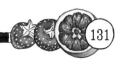
Simple Brown Rice Pilaf

1 cup brown rice
½ cup chopped onion
1 garlic clove, minced
2¼ cups reduced-sodium fat-free chicken
    broth

Nutrition Facts	
Serving Size ½ cup	
Servings Per Recipe 8	
Amount Per Serving	
Calories 95	
Total Fat 1g	
Cholesterol 0mg	
Sodium 162mg	
Total Carbohydrate 19g	
Dietary Fiber 1g	
Sugars 1g	
Protein 2g	

1. In 2 to 3-quart saucepan over medium heat, cook and stir rice, onion and garlic until rice is brown and onion is tender.

2. Stir in broth and bring to a boil. Reduce heat to low and simmer, covered, about 1 hour.

3. Remove from heat and let stand, covered, about 5 minutes. Fluff with fork.

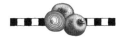

The simple, "new" carb rule: "If it's white, don't bite." "Bad" carbs are generally white in color, like sugar, white flour, and white bread.

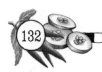

Carrot Brown Rice Pilaf

1 cup finely chopped onion
2 cups shredded carrots
¼ cup pine nuts
2 cups cooked brown rice

1. In sprayed nonstick 10 to 12-inch skillet over medium heat, cook and stir onion, carrots and pine nuts until onions are tender.

2. Stir in brown rice and heat through.

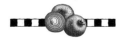

Nutrition Facts
Serving Size ½ cup
Servings Per Recipe 8
Amount Per Serving
Calories 88
Total Fat 2g
Cholesterol 0mg
Sodium 20mg
Total Carbohydrate 16g
Dietary Fiber 2g
Sugars 2g
Protein 2g

Brown rice is used in most of the rice recipes, and the nutty flavor and somewhat chewy texture of brown rice complements many vegetable combinations. Keep brown rice in the freezer to keep it fresh for cooking.

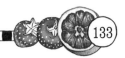

Curried Brown Rice

1 cup finely chopped onion
½ - 1 teaspoon curry powder
2 cups cooked brown rice
⅓ cup golden raisins

1. In sprayed nonstick 10 to 12-inch skillet over medium heat, cook and stir onions until tender.

2. Add curry powder and cook for about 30 seconds. Stir in brown rice and raisins and heat through.

Nutrition Facts	
Serving Size ½ cup	
Servings Per Recipe 8	
Amount Per Serving	
Calories 82	
Total Fat 0g	
Cholesterol 0mg	
Sodium 2mg	
Total Carbohydrate 18g	
Dietary Fiber 2g	
Sugars 4g	
Protein 2g	

Curry powder, widely used in Indian cooking, is a blend of 20 different spices. Use sparingly and, for best flavor, keep stored, airtight, no longer than 2 months.

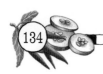

Poblano Chilies with Cheese

2 medium poblano chilies
1 cup reduced-fat cottage cheese, drained
¼ cup chopped green onion
½ cup reduced-fat colby Jack cheese

Nutrition Facts	
Serving Size ½ chile	
Servings Per Recipe 4	
Amount Per Serving	
Calories 49	
Total Fat 1g	
Cholesterol 2mg	
Sodium 211mg	
Total Carbohydrate 3g	
Dietary Fiber 0g	
Sugars 1g	
Protein 7g	

1. Preheat broiler.

2. Split poblano chilies with sharp knife and remove seeds, but leave stems on. Rinse and pat dry on paper towels.

3. On foil-covered baking sheet, 4 to 5 inches from heat, broil chilies on all sides until skin chars.

4. Remove and seal in plastic bag``. When cool, carefully peel skin away.

5. Preheat oven to 350°.

6. Arrange chilies in sprayed 9 x 9-inch baking dish. Spoon cottage cheese into chilies and sprinkle with green onions and cheese.

7. Bake 15 to 20 minutes or until cheese melts.

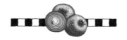

How hot are poblano chilies as compared to jalapeño chilies? The ever-popular jalapeño chilies are over 2 times hotter than poblano chilies. If you aren't into hot, you'll be pleased with the milder flavor of poblanos.

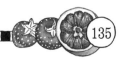

Green Chile Cheese Bake

2 (4 ounce) cans whole green chilies
1½ cups shredded reduced-fat Mexican
    cheese, divided
¾ cup liquid egg substitute
½ cup fat-free milk

Nutrition Facts	
Serving Size ¾ cup	
Servings Per Recipe 6	
Amount Per Serving	
Calories 92	
Total Fat 4g	
Cholesterol 15mg	
Sodium 288mg	
Total Carbohydrate 4g	
Dietary Fiber 1g	
Sugars 2g	
Protein 9g	

1. Preheat oven to 350°.

2. Rinse green chilies, remove seeds and pat
   dry on paper towels. Spread whole chilies
   on bottom of sprayed 9 x 9-inch baking dish.
   Sprinkle ¾ cup cheese on top and add layer of
   remaining chilies.

3. Whisk egg substitute and milk and pour over green chilies.
   Sprinkle with remaining cheese. Bake 30 minutes.

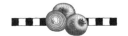

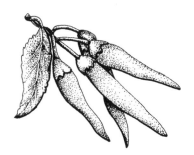

Meatless Fajita Bowl

1 (16 ounce) package frozen onion and bell
    pepper strips
2 cups frozen veggie crumbles (soy protein)
¼ cup reduced-fat sour cream
½ cup salsa

Nutrition Facts		
Serving Size 1 cup		
Servings Per Recipe 4		
Amount Per Serving		
Calories 126		
Total Fat 4g		
Cholesterol 10mg		
Sodium 265mg		
Total Carbohydrate 15g		
Dietary Fiber 4g		
Sugars 6g		
Protein 13g		

1. In sprayed nonstick 10 to 12-inch skillet over medium heat, cook and stir onions and peppers until tender. Add veggie crumbles and heat through.

2. Serve in bowls and top with sour cream and salsa.

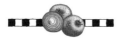

Check your supermarket to locate all the many soy products – veggie soy crumbles, taco filling, chorizo, burgers and soy "cheese" shreds. The products are found in refrigerated and freezer sections.

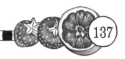
Pasta-Cheese Frittata

6 ounces reduced-carbohydrate spaghetti
1½ cups liquid egg substitute
1 tablespoon chopped green onion
1 cup shredded reduced-fat mozzarella cheese

Nutrition Facts	
Serving Size ⅛ frittata Servings Per Recipe 8	
Amount Per Serving	
Calories 113	
Total Fat 0g	
Cholesterol 0mg	
Sodium 198mg	
Total Carbohydrate 17g	
Dietary Fiber 2g	
Sugars 2g	
Protein 12g	

1. Preheat oven to 350°.

2. Cook pasta according to package directions. Drain well. Spoon into sprayed 9-inch pie plate.

3. Mix egg substitute, onion and cheese. Pour over spaghetti. Bake 30 minutes or until set. Cut into 8 wedges.

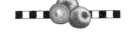

When shopping for grain products, you will find them described as refined, enriched and whole grain. Refined foods may have lost many nutrients in processing; enriched products have added iron, thiamin, riboflavin, niacin and folate. Whole grain products are rich in all nutrients found in the original grain.

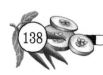

Soy Veggie Quesadillas

4 (6-inch) reduced-carbohydrate whole wheat
    tortillas
2 tablespoons soy veggie taco filling, divided
2 tablespoons salsa, divided
4 tablespoons shredded reduced-fat colby Jack
    cheese, divided

Nutrition Facts		
Serving Size 2 quesadilla wedges Servings Per Recipe 4		
Amount Per Serving		
Calories 55		
Total Fat 2g		
Cholesterol 0mg		
Sodium 228mg		
Total Carbohydrate 7g		
Dietary Fiber 5g		
Sugars 1g		
Protein 3g		

1. For each quesadilla, spread 1 tortilla with
    1 tablespoon taco filling, 1 tablespoon salsa
    and 2 tablespoons cheese. Top with another
    tortilla. Repeat for second quesadilla.

2. Preheat sprayed nonstick 12-inch skillet or
    griddle on medium-high heat. Use a spatula to place quesadilla
    in skillet.

3. Cook for 2 minutes on each side or until filling is hot and cheese
    melts. Remove with spatula and cut each quesadilla into 4 wedges.

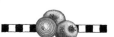

*Soybean products, unlike some other beans, offer
a "complete protein" – one that contains all the
essential proteins for body needs. Animal-based
foods also have complete protein but generally offer
more fat, especially saturated fat.*

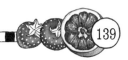
Veggie Frittata

½ cup chopped broccoli florets
¼ cup shredded carrots
1½ cups liquid egg substitute
1 cup shredded reduced-fat cheddar cheese

1. Preheat oven to 350°.

2. In sprayed nonstick 6 to 8-inch skillet over medium-high heat, cook and stir broccoli and carrots about 2 minutes or until tender. Transfer to sprayed 9-inch pie plate.

3. Mix egg substitute and cheese and pour over vegetables in pie plate. Bake 30 to 40 minutes or until set. Cut into 6 wedges.

Nutrition Facts		
Serving Size ⅙ frittata Servings Per Recipe 6		
Amount Per Serving		
Calories 60		
Total Fat 0g		
Cholesterol 0mg		
Sodium 266mg		
Total Carbohydrate 3g		
Dietary Fiber 1g		
Sugars 2g		
Protein 12g		

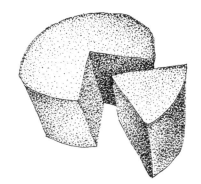

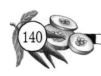

Cannellini Beans and Greens

1 cup chopped onion
1 (15½ ounce) can cannellini beans (white
    kidney beans) with liquid
3 cups fresh baby spinach
1 tablespoon lemon juice

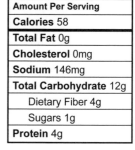

Nutrition Facts
Serving Size ½ cup
Servings Per Recipe 7
Amount Per Serving
Calories 58
Total Fat 0g
Cholesterol 0mg
Sodium 146mg
Total Carbohydrate 12g
Dietary Fiber 4g
Sugars 1g
Protein 4g

1. In sprayed nonstick 10 to 12-inch skillet,
    cook and stir onion until tender. Add beans
    and ½ cup water.

2. Bring to a boil, stir in spinach and cook
    just until spinach wilts. Sprinkle with
    lemon juice.

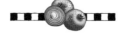

> *If you're looking to reduce calories, cannellini
> beans – 90 calories per ½ cup – are a better choice
> than navy beans at 148 calories per ½ cup.*

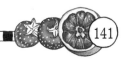
Portobello Pizza

1 cup thinly sliced baby portobello (2-inch)
    mushrooms
3 tablespoons fat-free balsamic vinaigrette
    dressing
1 (7 x 8-inch) thin roll-up whole grain flatbread
⅓ cup shredded reduced-fat mozzarella cheese

Nutrition Facts	
Serving Size ¼ flatbread	
Servings Per Recipe 4	
Amount Per Serving	
Calories 54	
Total Fat 1g	
Cholesterol 2mg	
Sodium 180mg	
Total Carbohydrate 6g	
Dietary Fiber 2g	
Sugars 1g	
Protein 7g	

1. Preheat oven to 450°.

2. Marinate mushrooms in dressing in plastic
    bag for 10 minutes.

3. Place flatbread on sprayed foil-lined baking
    pan. Spread with mushrooms and cheese.

4. Bake for 5 to 7 minutes or just until mushrooms are tender and
    cheese melts. Cut in fourths.

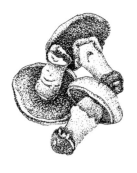

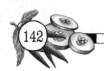

Tomato-Mozzarella Flatbread

1 (7 x 8-inch) thin roll-up whole grain flatbread
⅓ cup shredded reduced-fat mozzarella cheese
1 medium tomato, thinly sliced
1 teaspoon olive oil

Nutrition Facts		
Serving Size ¼ flatbread Servings Per Recipe 2		
Amount Per Serving		
Calories 66		
Total Fat 3g		
Cholesterol 2mg		
Sodium 137mg		
Total Carbohydrate 6g		
Dietary Fiber 2g		
Sugar 2g		
Protein 5g		

1. Preheat oven to 400°.

2. Place flatbread on sprayed foil-lined baking pan. Sprinkle with cheese and arrange tomato slices on top. Drizzle with olive oil.

3. Bake for about 5 minutes or until cheese melts. Cut into fourths.

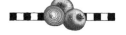

Can diabetics eat only small amounts of bread, potatoes and pasta? These foods are part of a healthy meal plan, but portion size is the key. Follow your recommended meal plan to determine how much and how often you can eat these foods.

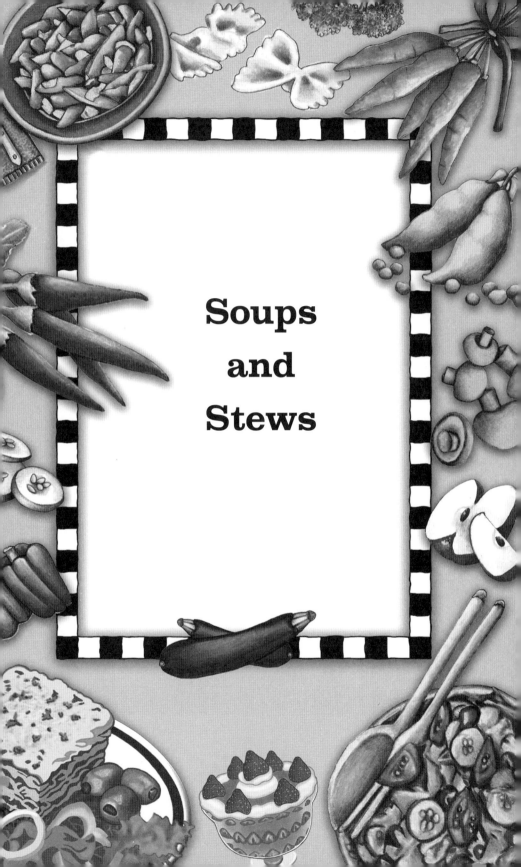

Soups
and
Stews

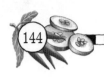

Soups and Stews Contents

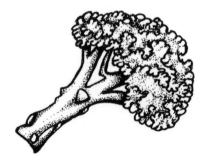

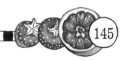
Creamy Broccoli Soup

3 cups "Sally's Seasoning Blend" (garlic, onion,
    bell pepper, celery), p. 217
5 cups coarsely chopped broccoli florets
1 (32 ounce) carton reduced-sodium fat-free
    chicken broth
¼ cup fat-free half-and-half cream

Nutrition Facts		
Serving Size 1 cup		
Servings Per recipe 8		
Amount Per Serving		
Calories 63		
Total Fat 0g		
Cholesterol 0mg		
Sodium 327mg		
Total Carbohydrate 9g		
Dietary Fiber 3g		
Sugars 4g		
Protein 4g		

1. In sprayed large, heavy pan over medium-high
    heat, cook and stir onion mixture until tender.

2. Stir in florets and broth, and bring to a boil.

3. Reduce heat and slowly boil until broccoli is
    soft enough to mash.

4. Cool about 10 minutes. Transfer in batches to food processor or
    blender and process until smooth.

5. Return to pan, pour in cream and heat slowly.

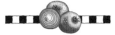

*How much broccoli to buy? 1 pound of broccoli
yields 5 to 6 cups florets and sliced stems.*

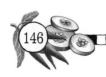

Spinach-Egg Soup

2 (14 ounce) cans reduced-sodium fat-free
    chicken broth
1 (10 ounce) package washed baby spinach
1 hard-cooked egg, chopped
2 tablespoons grated parmesan cheese

1. Bring broth to boiling in large, heavy pan over
    medium-high heat. Reduce heat to simmer.

2. Stir in spinach just until it wilts. Garnish
    servings with chopped egg and parmesan cheese.

Nutrition Facts	
Serving Size 1 cup	
Servings Per Recipe 4	
Amount Per Serving	
Calories 53	
Total Fat 2g	
Cholesterol 57mg	
Sodium 403mg	
Total Carbohydrate 2g	
Dietary Fiber 1g	
Sugars 1g	
Protein 6g	

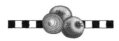

Zesty Tomato Soup

1 (46 ounce) bottle reduced-sodium
    vegetable juice
1 teaspoon dried basil, crushed
⅛ - ¼ teaspoon ground red pepper
¼ teaspoon garlic powder

1. Pour vegetable juice in 2-quart saucepan.
    Stir in basil, red pepper and garlic powder.

2. Bring to a boil, reduce heat and simmer
    about 5 minutes.

Nutrition Facts	
Serving Size 1 cup	
Servings Per Recipe 6	
Amount Per Serving	
Calories 51	
Total Fat 0g	
Cholesterol 0mg	
Sodium 140mg	
Total Carbohydrate 10g	
Dietary Fiber 2g	
Sugars 8g	
Protein 2g	

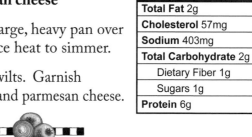

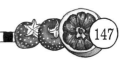
Butternut Squash Soup

1 (2 pound) butternut squash, peeled,
   seeded, cut in 2-inch pieces
3 cups reduced-sodium vegetarian vegetable
   broth
¼ teaspoon dried thyme, crushed
¼ cup fat-free half-and-half cream

Nutrition Facts		
Serving Size 1 cup		
Servings Per Recipe About 3		
Amount Per Serving		
Calories 86		
Total Fat 0g		
Cholesterol 0mg		
Sodium 476mg		
Total Carbohydrate 20g		
Dietary Fiber 3g		
Sugars 5g		
Protein 2g		

1. In large, heavy pan over medium high
   heat, bring vegetable broth to a boil and
   add squash and thyme.

2. Boil slowly until squash is very soft, about
   20 minutes. Cool about 10 minutes.

3. Transfer to food processor or blender and process until smooth.
   Return to pan, stir cream and heat slowly.

4. Number of servings will vary due to loss of liquid during cooking.

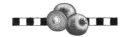

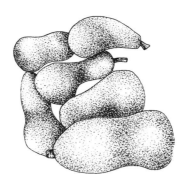

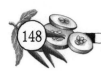
Cauliflower-Cheese Soup

1 cup chopped onion
3 (14 ounce) cans reduced-sodium fat-free
   chicken broth
5 cups cauliflower small florets
½ cup shredded reduced fat cheddar cheese

Nutrition Facts	
Serving Size 1 cup	
Servings Per Recipe 8	
Amount Per Serving	
Calories 44	
Total Fat 1g	
Cholesterol 0mg	
Sodium 628mg	
Total Carbohydrate 6g	
Dietary Fiber 2g	
Sugars 3g	
Protein 4g	

1. Cook and stir onions until tender in sprayed large, heavy pan over medium heat.

2. Add broth and florets, and bring to a boil. Reduce heat, cover and simmer until cauliflower is tender, about 20 minutes. Cool for about 10 minutes.

3. Transfer in batches to food processor or blender and process until smooth. Garnish with cheese.

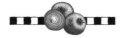

"After all the trouble you go to, you get about as much actual "food" out of eating an artichoke as you would from licking 30 or 40 postage stamps."
                                –Miss Piggy

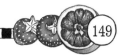
Golden Onion Soup

6 medium yellow onions, thinly sliced
¼ teaspoon dried thyme
2 tablespoons sherry cooking wine or dry sherry
4 (4 gram) packets sodium-free beef broth
    seasoning

Nutrition Facts		
Serving Size 1 cup		
Servings Per Recipe 6		
Amount Per Serving		
Calories 51		
Total Fat 0g		
Cholesterol 0mg		
Sodium 38mg		
Total Carbohydrate 12g		
Dietary Fiber 2g		
Sugars 5g		
Protein 1g		

1. In sprayed, large heavy pan over medium
    heat, cook and stir onions and thyme about
    15 minutes or until the onions begin to
    brown.

2. Reduce heat to low and cook onions, stirring
    more often, about 25 minutes or until onions
    turn a rich brown color.

3. Add wine and heat to a boil until wine evaporates. Stir in 4 cups
    water and broth packets and bring to a boil.

4. Reduce heat and simmer about 25 minutes.

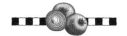

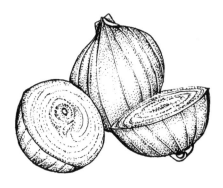

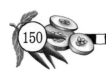

Home-Style Lentil Soup

3 cups "Sally's Seasoning Blend" (garlic, onion,
  celery, bell pepper), p. 217
1 cup chopped carrots
1 cup dried brown lentils, rinsed, drained
1 teaspoon dried oregano, crushed

Nutrition Facts
Serving Size 1 cup
Servings Per Recipe 10
Amount Per Serving
Calories 63
Total Fat 0g
Cholesterol 0mg
Sodium 27mg
Total Carbohydrate 14g
Dietary Fiber 6g
Sugars 4g
Protein 5g

1. In sprayed nonstick large, heavy pan on
    medium heat, cook and stir onion mixture
    and carrots until tender, about 6 to 8 minutes.

2. Add lentils, oregano, and 6 cups water. Bring
    to a boil.

3. Reduce heat, cover, and simmer about 50 to 60 minutes or until
    lentils are tender.

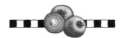

> *Have you wondered what "legumes" are? Plants
> of the bean and pea family, with seeds that are rich
> in protein, as compared to other plant foods. Legumes
> include black beans, garbanzo beans, black-eyed peas,
> kidney beans, lentils, soybeans and peanuts.*

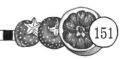
Louisiana Vegetable Soup

1 (12 ounce) package frozen chopped onion,
    celery, bell pepper, parsley blend
1 (14 ounce) can reduced-sodium fat-free
    chicken broth
1 (14½ ounce) can diced tomatoes with basil,
    garlic and oregano
1 (16 ounce) package frozen cut okra

Nutrition Facts	
Serving Size 1 cup	
Servings Per Recipe 4	
Amount Per Serving	
Calories 86	
Total Fat 0g	
Cholesterol 0mg	
Sodium 663mg	
Total Carbohydrate 17g	
Dietary Fiber 4g	
Sugars 6g	
Protein 4g	

1. In sprayed large, heavy pan on medium-high
   heat, cook and stir onion mixture until tender.

2. Pour in broth and tomatoes and bring to a
   boil. Add okra, reduce heat to medium and
   simmer uncovered for 15 to 20 minutes or until okra is tender.

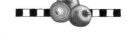

Fresh okra is popular across the South, whether fried, stewed with tomatoes or added to soups. Although many folks don't like the viscous substance released when okra is cooked, it is used in gumbos for both thickening and flavoring.

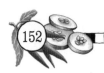

Roasted Red Pepper Soup

4 medium red bell peppers
1 cup chopped onion
5 cups reduced-sodium vegetable broth
¼ cup fat-free half-and-half cream

Nutrition Facts	
Serving Size 1 cup	
Servings Per Recipe 6	
Amount Per Serving	
Calories 50	
Total Fat 0g	
Cholesterol 0mg	
Sodium 389mg	
Total Carbohydrate 10g	
Dietary Fiber 2g	
Sugars 6g	
Protein 1g	

1. Preheat broiler and line broiler pan with foil. Place peppers on pan and broil 4 to 5 inches from heat, turning frequently, until skins are charred.

2. Seal peppers in plastic bag. When cool, peel skin from peppers and cut in half.

3. Discard seeds and membrane and coarsely chop peppers.

4. Cook and stir onion until tender in sprayed large, heavy pan over medium high heat. Stir in roasted peppers and broth and bring to a boil.

5. Reduce heat to simmer and cook until peppers become tender, about 10 minutes.

6. Remove pan from heat and cool about 5 minutes. Transfer soup in batches to food processor or blender and process until smooth. Return soup to pan, stir in cream and heat slowly.

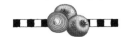

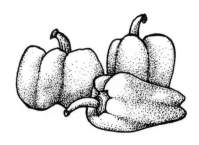

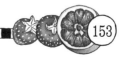

Spicy Cabbage Soup

2 cups finely chopped onion
1 (14 ounce) diced tomatoes with green chilies
1 (8 ounce) can no-salt tomato sauce
3 cups shredded green cabbage

Nutrition Facts	
Serving Size 1 cup Servings Per Recipe 6	
Amount Per Serving	
Calories 50	
Total Fat 0g	
Cholesterol 0mg	
Sodium 350mg	
Total Carbohydrate 10g	
Dietary Fiber 3g	
Sugars 6g	
Protein 2g	

1. In sprayed large, heavy pan over medium heat, cook and stir onions until tender.

2. Process tomatoes in blender or food processor about 30 seconds. Stir tomatoes, tomato sauce and 4 cups water into pan with onions.

3. Bring to a boil, reduce heat and simmer, uncovered, about 15 minutes. Stir in cabbage and cook until just tender.

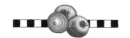

To measure liquid ingredients, place a glass measuring cup on a level work surface and add the desired amount of liquid. Bend down to check the accuracy of the measure at eye level. Angled measuring cups allow you to check the amount from above.

Veggie Crumble Chili

1 (16 ounce) package frozen chopped onion,
   celery, bell pepper and parsley blend
1 (12 ounce) package veggie protein crumbles
1 (14½ ounce) can no-salt-added stewed
   tomatoes
2 - 3 teaspoons chili powder

Nutrition Facts
Serving Size ¾ cup
Servings Per Recipe 4
Amount Per Serving
Calories 144
Total Fat 1g
Cholesterol 0mg
Sodium 464mg
Total Carbohydrate 20g
Dietary Fiber 7g
Sugars 6g
Protein 21g

1. Cook and stir onion mixture about 8 minutes or until tender in sprayed nonstick large, heavy pan on medium heat.

2. Add crumbles, tomatoes and chili powder. Bring to a boil, reduce heat and simmer about 10 minutes.

Add black beans to your eating repertoire to reap the rewards of healthy protein, antioxidants and fiber.

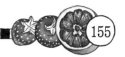
Slow Cooker Ground Beef Soup

1 medium onion, chopped
1 pound 90% lean ground beef
1 (16 ounce) package frozen soup vegetables
2 (14½ ounce) cans Italian stewed tomatoes

Nutrition Facts		
Serving Size 1 cup		
Servings Per Recipe 12		
Amount Per Serving		
Calories 105		
Total Fat 4g		
Cholesterol 3mg		
Sodium 151mg		
Total Carbohydrate 7g		
Dietary Fiber 2g		
Sugars 3g		
Protein 9g		

1. Cook and stir onion until tender in sprayed nonstick 10 to 12-inch skillet. Remove and add ground beef. Brown beef and drain.

2. Pour soup vegetables and onion in bottom of 4 to 5-quart slow cooker. Add ground beef, tomatoes and 2½ cups water. Cover and cook on LOW for 4 to 6 hours.

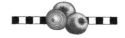

A slow cooker must be at least half full and no more than two-thirds full. Resist lifting the lid of the slow cooker – lost heat is not quickly recovered due to the low cooking temperatures.

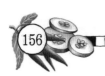

Slow Cooker Beef Stew

2 pounds lean beef roast, trimmed, cut in
   1-inch cubes
1 (16 ounce) package frozen pearl onions
3 carrots, peeled, cut in 2-inch pieces
1 (14½ ounce) can diced fire-roasted tomatoes
   with garlic

Nutrition Facts
Serving Size 1 cup
Servings Per Recipe 8
Amount Per Serving
Calories 211
Total Fat 6g
Cholesterol 61mg
Sodium 133mg
Total Carbohydrate 11g
Dietary Fiber 2g
Sugars 7g
Protein 26g

1. Brown beef cubes in sprayed nonstick 10 to
   12-inch skillet.

2. Layer onions and carrots in slow cooker.
   Add beef cubes and pour in tomatoes. Cover
   and cook on LOW 6 to 8 hours.

3. Check beef for tenderness. If needed, continue cooking
   for 1 to 2 hours or until beef becomes very tender.

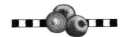

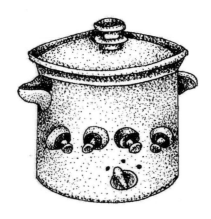

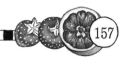

Beefy Vegetable Stew

1 pound 90% lean ground beef
1 (14½ ounce) can diced tomatoes with basil,
    garlic and oregano
1 (16 ounce) package frozen stew vegetables
1 (4g) packet sodium-free beef bouillon

1. In sprayed nonstick 10 to 12-inch skillet,
   brown beef. Drain and transfer to sprayed
   4 to 5-quart slow cooker.

2. Pour in tomatoes, stew vegetables, 1 cup
   water and bouillon. Stir, cover and cook on
   LOW for 4 to 6 hours.

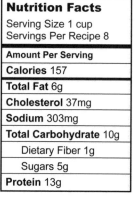

Nutrition Facts	
Serving Size 1 cup	
Servings Per Recipe 8	
Amount Per Serving	
Calories 157	
Total Fat 6g	
Cholesterol 37mg	
Sodium 303mg	
Total Carbohydrate 10g	
Dietary Fiber 1g	
Sugars 5g	
Protein 13g	

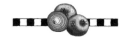

*What is the benefit of browning when meats will
be cooked in a slow cooker? Browning adds flavor
and color and helps keep moisture on the inside.*

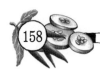

Lean Beef Chili

1 cup finely chopped onion
1 (1 pound) package 90% lean ground beef
1 (10 ounce) can diced tomatoes and
    green chilies
1 tablespoon chili powder

Nutrition Facts		
Serving Size 1 cup		
Servings Per Recipe 4		
Amount Per Serving		
Calories 234		
Total Fat 12g		
Cholesterol 74mg		
Sodium 421mg		
Total Carbohydrate 7g		
Dietary Fiber 2g		
Sugars 4g		
Protein 24g		

1. Cook and stir onion until tender in sprayed nonstick 10 to 12-inch skillet over medium heat. Do not brown. Remove from skillet.

2. Add beef to skillet, cook and stir over medium heat until it browns. Drain beef and return to skillet.

3. Stir in onion, tomatoes and chili powder. Add 1 to 2 cups water and simmer 25 to 30 minutes.

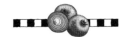

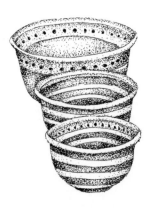

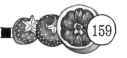

Skinny Chicken Gumbo Soup

2 (14 ounce) cans reduced-sodium fat-free
    chicken broth
1 (16 ounce) package frozen sliced bell peppers
    and onions
1 (16 ounce) package frozen sliced okra
2 cups chopped cooked chicken breast

1. Bring broth and 1 cup water to a boil in large, heavy pan. Add frozen vegetables.

2. Reduce heat to medium and cook until vegetables are tender. Reduce heat to low, add chicken and simmer about 5 minutes.

Nutrition Facts	
Serving Size 1 cup	
Servings Per Recipe 8	
Amount Per Serving	
Calories 91	
Total Fat 1g	
Cholesterol 27mg	
Sodium 183mg	
Total Carbohydrate 7g	
Dietary Fiber 2g	
Sugars 3g	
Protein 12g	

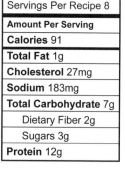

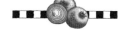

Soy products, such as green edamame and roasted soy nuts, contain complex carbohydrates, protein and heart-healthy fat.

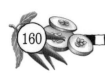

Speedy Chicken Vegetable Soup

1 cup frozen chopped onion, celery, bell pepper
    and parsley blend
3 (14 ounce) cans reduced-sodium fat-free
    chicken broth
1 (10 ounce) package frozen mixed vegetables
    (corn, carrots, peas, green beans)
2 cups chopped cooked chicken breast

Nutrition Facts	
Serving Size 1 cup	
Servings Per Recipe 8	
Amount Per Serving	
Calories 97	
Total Fat 1g	
Cholesterol 27mg	
Sodium 476mg	
Total Carbohydrate 7g	
Dietary Fiber 3g	
Sugars 1g	
Protein 14g	

1. In sprayed large, heavy pan, cook and stir onion mixture until tender. Add chicken broth and bring to a boil.

2. Stir frozen mixed vegetables into broth and return to boiling.

3. Reduce heat to slow boil and continue cooking for about 6 minutes or until vegetables become tender. Stir in chicken.

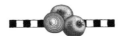

According to experts, moderate physical activity helps control diabetes. Studies have also found that moderate physical activity even reduced the risk of developing diabetes by more than half.

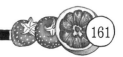
Chicken Oriental Soup

1 (32 ounce) carton reduced-sodium fat-free
    chicken broth
1 tablespoon reduced-sodium soy sauce
1 cup shredded cooked chicken breast
2 tablespoons chopped green onion

1. Bring broth and soy sauce to boiling in
   3 to 4-quart saucepan. Add chicken,
   reduce heat, cook about 5 minutes and stir
   in onions.

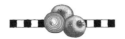

Nutrition Facts		
Serving Size 1 cup		
Servings Per Recipe About 5		
Amount Per Serving		
Calories 48		
Total Fat 1g		
Cholesterol 18mg		
Sodium 491mg		
Total Carbohydrate 1g		
Dietary Fiber 0g		
Sugars 1g		
Protein 9g		

Do you drink enough water? At least 8 to 10 glasses of water and other liquids daily are recommended. Beverages such as milk and tea count, but remember that water is the best thirst quencher.

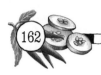

Chicken Noodle Soup

1 (32 ounce) carton reduced-sodium fat-free
   chicken broth
1 medium carrot, sliced
½ cup uncooked medium egg noodles
1 cup chopped, cooked chicken

1. Bring broth to a boil in 2 to 3-quart
   saucepan. Add carrot, reduce heat to
   medium, and cook until carrot is tender.

2. Increase heat to boiling and stir in noodles.
   Reduce heat to medium and cook 10 minutes
   or until noodles are tender. Stir in chicken.

Nutrition Facts
Serving Size 1 cup
Servings Per Recipe 6
Amount Per Serving
Calories 118
Total Fat 2g
Cholesterol 31mg
Sodium 601mg
Total Carbohydrate 15g
Dietary Fiber 1g
Sugars 1g
Protein 10g

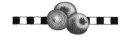

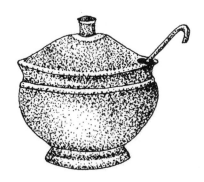

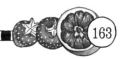

Italian Sausage and Zucchini Soup

1 pound Italian turkey sausage, casings
    removed, crumbled
1 (14 ounce) can no-salt-added stewed tomatoes
3 (14 ounce) cans reduced-sodium fat-free
    chicken broth
3 medium zucchini, cut in ½-inch pieces

Nutrition Facts	
Serving Size 1 cup	
Servings Per Recipe 6	
Amount Per Serving	
Calories 164	
Total Fat 7g	
Cholesterol 46mg	
Sodium 667mg	
Total Carbohydrate 9g	
Dietary Fiber 2g	
Sugars 7g	
Protein 15g	

1. In sprayed large, heavy pan over medium-high
   heat, cook and stir sausage until it browns,
   about 8 minutes.

2. Pour in tomatoes and chicken broth. Bring to
   a boil, reduce heat and simmer, covered, about
   10 minutes.

3. Add zucchini and simmer, covered, about 20 minutes or until
   zucchini is tender.

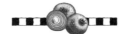

    *The 2-hour rule for food safety is to refrigerate
or freeze food within 2 hours from the minute it
comes out of the oven or refrigerator. This includes
food preparation and serving time.*

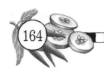

Southwest Pork Stew

1 pound boneless pork shoulder roast, cut in
    ¾ inch cubes
3 cups "Sally's Seasoning Blend" (garlic,
    onions, bell peppers, celery), p. 217
1 (10 ounce) can diced tomatoes and
    green chilies
1 (15½ ounce) can yellow hominy, rinsed,
    drained

Nutrition Facts	
Serving Size ¾ cup	
Servings Per Recipe 6	
Amount Per Serving	
Calories 148	
Total Fat 4g	
Cholesterol 38mg	
Sodium 450mg	
Total Carbohydrate 11g	
Dietary Fiber 1g	
Sugars 3g	
Protein 12g	

1. In sprayed nonstick large, heavy pan, brown pork cubes on all sides. Remove from pan.

2. Add onion mixture to pan; cook and stir on medium heat until vegetables become tender.

3. Add tomatoes and pork cubes and bring to a boil. Reduce heat to simmer and cook, covered, about 40 minutes or until pork becomes very tender.

4. Add hominy, heat through and serve.

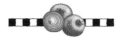

A food weight scale to measure ounces and pounds is a good investment for accurate measurements.

Main Dishes

Beef
Chicken and Turkey
Pork
Seafood

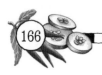

Main Dishes Contents

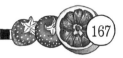

Beefy Ramen Noodles

1 (3 ounce) package ramen noodles
1 pound 90% lean ground beef
1 medium red or green bell pepper, chopped
1 (14½ ounce) can diced tomatoes with
    roasted garlic

Nutrition Facts	
Serving Size ¾ cup Servings Per Recipe 8	
Amount Per Serving	
Calories 163	
Total Fat 7g	
Cholesterol 5mg	
Sodium 486mg	
Total Carbohydrate 10g	
Dietary Fiber 1g	
Sugars 2g	
Protein 13g	

1. Cook noodles according to package directions. Discard seasoning packet. Rinse and drain noodles.

2. Brown ground beef in nonstick 10 to 12-inch skillet over medium-high heat. Remove beef and drain.

3. To same skillet, add bell peppers and cook and stir over medium heat 3 to 4 minutes or until tender.

4. Add tomatoes, beef and noodles to skillet. Cook and stir over medium heat 2 to 3 minutes.

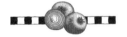

Take time to enjoy every moment of your meals at home. Eating on the run can limit your healthy food choices.

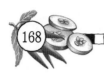

■ ■

Southwest Hamburgers

Nutrition Facts
Serving Size 1 patty
Servings Per Recipe 4
Amount Per Serving
Calories 228
Total Fat 11g
Cholesterol 74mg
Sodium 203mg
Total Carbohydrate 6g
Dietary Fiber 2g
Sugars 4g
Protein 24g

1 pound 90% lean ground beef
1 medium onion, thinly sliced
2 medium bell peppers (red and yellow or green), thinly sliced
4 tablespoons salsa

1. Divide beef into 4 patties and grill or broil until done.

2. In sprayed nonstick 10 to 12-inch skillet on medium heat, cook and stir onion and bell peppers until tender.

3. Serve beef patties topped with bell pepper-onion mixture and 1 tablespoon salsa.

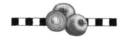

Ground beef will last one to two days in the refrigerator; after that, put it in the freezer.

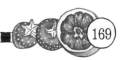

Slow Cooker Chuck Roast

1 (2 pound) boneless beef chuck roast,
    trimmed
1 cup chopped onion
2 garlic cloves, minced
¼ cup cider vinegar

Nutrition Facts		
Serving Size 4 ounces		
Servings Per Recipe 6 to 8		
Amount Per Serving		
Calories 170		
Total Fat 6g		
Cholesterol 61mg		
Sodium 85mg		
Total Carbohydrate 2g		
Dietary Fiber 0g		
Sugars 1g		
Protein 25g		

1. Brown roast on all sides in sprayed large, heavy pan on medium-high heat. Transfer to 4 to 5-quart slow cooker.

2. Add onion to pan and cook, over medium heat, until tender. Add garlic and cook about 30 seconds.

3. Stir in vinegar and scrape browned bits from pan. Pour ¼ cup water and vinegar mixture over roast

4. Cover and cook on LOW for 10 to 12 hours or until tender.

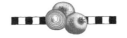

    An accepted rule is to salt most cuts of meat after cooking to keep their juiciness, except for roasts. Salting a roast actually adds flavor as it cooks without drying it out.

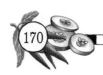

Slow Cooker Swiss Steak

1 pound beef cubed steaks
1 medium onion, cut in strips
1 medium green bell pepper, cut in strips
1 (14½ ounce) can roasted diced tomatoes
  with garlic

Nutrition Facts
Serving Size 4 ounce steak with vegetables
Servings Per Recipe 4
Amount Per Serving
Calories 209
Total Fat 8g
Cholesterol 69mg
Sodium 91mg
Total Carbohydrate 8g
Dietary Fiber 2g
Sugars 5g
Protein 25

1. In sprayed nonstick 10 to 12-inch skillet over medium-high heat, brown cubed beef steaks. Remove from skillet and reduce heat to medium.

2. Add onion and bell pepper strips and cook and stir 4 to 5 minutes or until tender.

3. Place onion and bell pepper strips in slow cooker and arrange steaks on top. Pour tomatoes over steaks. Cover and cook on LOW for 6 to 8 hours.

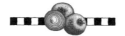

When handling raw meat, wash your hands in hot, soapy water before and after handling meat. Wash all surfaces and utensils in hot, soapy water after contact with raw meat. If you are grilling, don't serve cooked meat on the unwashed platter used to carry it to the grill.

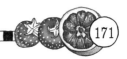
Beef Fajita Pitas

8 ounces flank steak, trimmed

3 tablespoons "Beef Fajita Marinade," p. 225

1 (16 ounce) package frozen bell pepper and
    onion strips, thawed

2 (4 inch) whole wheat pita breads

Nutrition Facts	
Serving Size 1 pita half	
Servings Per Recipe 4	
Amount Per Serving	
Calories 147	
Total Fat 4g	
Cholesterol 19mg	
Sodium 118mg	
Total Carbohydrate 14g	
Dietary Fiber 2g	
Sugars 4g	
Protein 15g	

1. Freeze meat for about 30 minutes. Slice thinly across grain into bite-size strips. Seal in plastic bag with marinade. Refrigerate for 2 to 4 hours. Drain.

2. Cook and stir vegetables until tender in sprayed nonstick 10 to 12-inch skillet over medium-high heat. Spray as needed. Remove from skillet.

3. Add beef to hot skillet, cook and stir about 2 to 3 minutes or until fork-tender. Do not overcook.

4. Return vegetables to skillet and heat through. Spoon mixture into pita bread and cut in half.

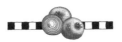

Is flank steak the same as skirt steak? No, but they come from the same general area of the beef — the flank or area between the ribs and hip. Flank is a long, thicker cut than skirt steak which is long but thinner. Both tend toward toughness and are usually marinated before cooking. Slow cooking produces more tender meat than fast cooking.

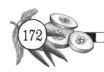

Fiesta Fajita Bowl

1 (16 ounce) package frozen grilled red and
    yellow peppers
1 pound boneless lean sirloin steak, cut in bite-
    size strips
½ cup frozen whole kernel corn, cooked
½ - ¾ cup salsa

Nutrition Facts	
Serving Size 1 cup	
Servings Per Recipe 4	
Amount Per Serving	
Calories 151	
Total Fat 3g	
Cholesterol 32mg	
Sodium 218mg	
Total Carbohydrate 10g	
Dietary Fiber 3g	
Sugars 6g	
Protein 18g	

1. Thaw peppers in microwave according to package instructions. Cut in strips and drain.

2. In sprayed nonstick 10 to 12-inch skillet on medium-high heat, cook and stir steak about 4 to 5 minutes, until just tender.

3. Add pepper strips, corn and salsa to skillet and heat through. Serve in bowls.

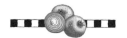

Weight Management: Drink a glass of water before you eat and another while you eat. Drink plenty of water throughout the day (8 glasses or more a day).

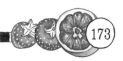
Baked Chicken and Broccoli

4 (4 ounce) boneless, skinless chicken breast
    halves (1 pound)
2 teaspoons olive oil
2 lemons, sliced
4 cups broccoli florets

Nutrition Facts	
Serving Size 1 chicken breast half with broccoli	
Servings Per Recipe 4	
Amount Per Serving	
Calories 191	
Total Fat 6g	
Cholesterol 73mg	
Sodium 163mg	
Total Carbohydrate 12g	
Dietary Fiber 5g	
Sugars 2g	
Protein 27g	

1. Preheat oven to 450°.

2. Rinse chicken breast halves and pat dry with paper towels. Rub chicken breast halves with olive oil.

3. Cut 4 (12-inch) squares of foil. Fold each square in half diagonally. Lay each breast to one side of diagonal crease.

4. Place 3 to 4 lemon slices on each chicken breast and top with 1 cup broccoli florets. Loosely fold foil over chicken and seal edges.

5. Bake for 15 minutes and check chicken breasts for doneness. (Be careful when opening steaming packets.)

6. If chicken is still pink, reseal and bake additional 5 to 6 minutes.

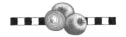

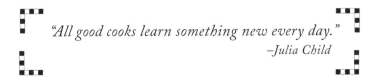

"All good cooks learn something new every day."
    –Julia Child

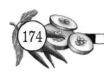

Baked Chicken Drumsticks

8 chicken drumsticks (1 pound)
1 tablespoon no-salt herb seasoning
3 - 4 tablespoons fresh lemon juice

Nutrition Facts		
Serving Size 1 drumstick		
Servings Per Recipe 8		
Amount Per Serving		
Calories 75		
Total Fat 2g		
Cholesterol 48mg		
Sodium 55mg		
Total Carbohydrate 0g		
Dietary Fiber 0g		
Sugars 0g		
Protein 13g		

1. Preheat oven to 350°. Use rubber gloves and kitchen shears to remove skin from drumsticks. Rinse and pat dry with paper towels.

2. Arrange drumsticks in sprayed 9 x 13-inch baking dish. Sprinkle both sides with herb seasoning.

3. Cover with foil and bake for 1 hour. Uncover and sprinkle with lemon juice.

4. Bake 15 minutes or until chicken is no longer pink.

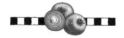

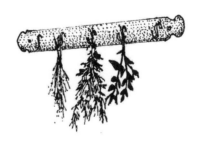

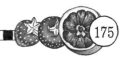

Skillet Chicken Breasts

4 (4 ounce) boneless skinless chicken breast
   halves (1 pound)
2 teaspoons dried rosemary, crushed
¼ cup cooking sherry or dry sherry
¼ cup fat-free reduced-sodium chicken broth

Nutrition Facts		
Serving Size 1 chicken breast half		
Servings Per Recipe 4		
Amount Per Serving		
Calories 145		
Total Fat 3g		
Cholesterol 76mg		
Sodium 264mg		
Total Carbohydrate 1g		
Dietary Fiber 0g		
Sugars 0g		
Protein 25g		

1. Rinse chicken breast halves and pat dry with
   paper towels.

2. Brown chicken on both sides in sprayed
   nonstick 10 to 12-inch skillet over
   medium heat.

3. Add rosemary, sherry and broth and bring
   to a boil. Reduce heat and simmer for about 30 minutes or until
   chicken is no longer pink.

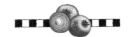

*When we gather at the dinner table, we form
bonds that translate into who we are and where
we come from. For one brief moment when we sit
down to enjoy a meal, carry on conversations and
listen to each other, we become a true family.*

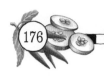

Sunny Mediterranean Chicken

4 (4 ounce) boneless skinless chicken breast
halves (1 pound)
1 (14½ ounce) can diced tomatoes with basil,
garlic, oregano
½ cup drained, sliced black olives
1 tablespoon finely grated lemon peel*

Nutrition Facts		
Serving Size 1 chicken breast half with sauce		
Servings Per Recipe 4		
Amount Per Serving		
Calories 193		
Total Fat 5g		
Cholesterol 73mg		
Sodium 322mg		
Total Carbohydrate 10g		
Dietary Fiber 2g		
Sugars 7g		
Protein 26g		

1. Rinse chicken and pat dry with paper towels.
   Heat sprayed nonstick 10 to 12-inch skillet
   on medium-high heat.

2. Add chicken, cover, and cook 5 to 7 minutes
   on each side or until no longer pink. Remove
   chicken from skillet.

3. Add tomatoes, olives and lemon peel to skillet. Cook and stir on
   medium heat about 4 minutes or until hot. Return chicken to
   skillet and heat through.

*TIP: Just grate the yellow peel and don't use any of the white pith. It is
too tart.

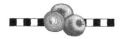

> The black olive, also known as Mission olive,
> is a ripe green olive that obtains its characteristic
> color and flavor from processing.

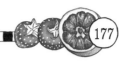
Greek-Style Baked Chicken

4 (4 ounce) boneless, skinless chicken breast
    halves (1 pound)
⅓ cup thinly sliced sun-dried tomatoes in oil
    plus 1 tablespoon oil
⅓ cup chopped ripe olives
⅓ cup grated parmesan cheese

Nutrition Facts		
Serving Size 1 chicken breast half with topping		
Servings Per Recipe 4		
Amount Per Serving		
Calories 202		
Total Fat 9g		
Cholesterol 78mg		
Sodium 384mg		
Total Carbohydrate 3g		
Dietary Fiber 1g		
Sugars 0g		
Protein 27g		

1. Preheat oven to 450°.

2. Rinse chicken and pat dry with paper towels. Rub chicken breast halves with oil from sun-dried tomatoes.

3. Cut 4 (12-inch) squares of foil. Fold each square in half diagonally. Lay each breast half to one side of crease.

4. Spoon 1 tablespoon tomatoes, 1 tablespoon olives and 1 tablespoon cheese on chicken. Loosely fold foil over chicken and seal edges.

5. Bake for 15 minutes and check chicken breasts for doneness. (Be careful when opening steaming packets.)

6. If chicken is still pink, reseal and bake about 5 minutes longer or until chicken is no longer pink.

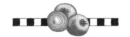

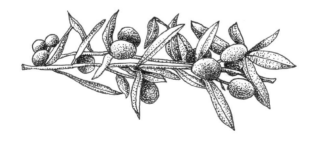

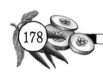

Spicy Stuffed Bell Peppers

2 red or yellow bell peppers, halved, seeded
¾ pound ground turkey breast
1 cup salsa
½ cup no-salt-added tomato sauce

Nutrition Facts	
Serving Size 1 stuffed pepper half	
Servings Per Recipe 4	
Amount Per Serving	
Calories 169	
Total Fat 2g	
Cholesterol 55mg	
Sodium 464mg	
Total Carbohydrate 10g	
Dietary Fiber 3g	
Sugars 6g	
Protein 28g	

1. Preheat oven to 350°.

2. Bring 3 quarts water to boil in a large heavy pan. Add pepper halves to boiling water and keep submerged for about 3 minutes. Drain and pat dry with paper towels.

3. Cook and stir turkey until no longer pink in sprayed nonstick 10 to 12-inch skillet on medium heat. Stir in salsa.

4. Stuff turkey-salsa mixture into pepper halves. Spoon 2 tablespoons tomato sauce on top and arrange in 9 x 9-inch baking dish.

5. Add ¼ cup water to dish and cover. Bake for 40 to 50 minutes.

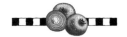

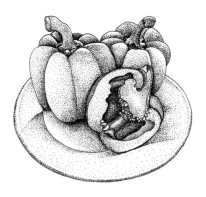

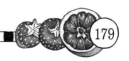
Slow Cooker Green Chile Chicken

1 pound boneless, skinless chicken thighs,
   fat removed
1 (16 ounce) package frozen onion and pepper
   strips, thawed
1 (10 ounce) can diced tomatoes and
   green chilies
½ teaspoon ground cumin

Nutrition Facts	
Serving Size 1 cup	
Servings Per Recipe 6	
Amount Per Serving	
Calories 120	
Total Fat 3g	
Cholesterol 63mg	
Sodium 290mg	
Total Carbohydrate 6g	
Dietary Fiber 1g	
Sugars 1g	
Protein 15g	

1. Rinse chicken thighs and pat dry with paper towels. Heat sprayed nonstick 10 to 12-inch skillet over medium-high heat and add thighs.

2. Brown one side of thighs, reduce heat to medium and brown other side; spray as needed. Remove from skillet.

3. Add onions and peppers to skillet and cook over medium heat until just tender.

4. Transfer onions and peppers to 4 to 5-quart slow cooker and arrange thighs on top. Pour in ¼ cup water and tomatoes.

5. Cook on LOW for 4 hours and stir in cumin. Cook additional 30 minutes or until thighs become very tender.

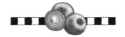

Transfer slow cooker leftovers to storage containers to refrigerate. If warm food is stored in the crockery liner in the refrigerator, the food may not cool down quickly enough to be safe to eat as leftovers.

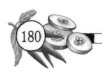

Chicken Quesadillas

¾ cup finely shredded colby Jack cheese, divided
½ cup shredded cooked chicken, divided
½ cup salsa, divided
3 (6 inch) flour tortillas

Nutrition Facts		
Serving Size ½ quesadilla		
Servings Per Recipe 6		
Amount Per Serving		
Calories 105		
Total Fat 4g		
Cholesterol 15mg		
Sodium 352mg		
Total Carbohydrate 9g		
Dietary Fiber 1g		
Sugars 2g		
Protein 8g		

1. Spread ¼ cup cheese, 2 tablespoons chicken and 2 tablespoons salsa over half of each tortilla. Fold tortillas in half.

2. In sprayed nonstick 10 to 12-inch skillet, cook quesadillas over medium heat for 3 to 4 minutes and turn once. Cut quesadillas in half to serve.

TIP: *In this recipe, you may want to substitute fat-free refried beans for the ½ cup chicken, although you need to be aware of the high sodium content of the canned beans.*

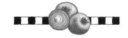

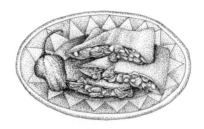

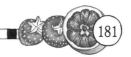
Fiesta Baked Chicken

4 (4 ounce) boneless, skinless chicken breast
    halves (1 pound)
⅓ cup thinly sliced sun-dried tomatoes in oil
    plus 1 tablespoon oil
½ cup drained diced green chilies
1 cup frozen whole kernel corn, thawed

Nutrition Facts		
Serving Size 1 chicken packet		
Servings Per Recipe 4		
Amount Per Serving		
Calories 183		
Total Fat 5g		
Cholesterol 73mg		
Sodium 226mg		
Total Carbohydrate 10g		
Dietary Fiber 2g		
Sugars 1g		
Protein 26g		

1. Preheat oven to 450°.

2. Rinse chicken and pat dry with paper towels.
    Rub chicken breast halves with 1 tablespoon
    oil from sun-dried tomatoes.

3. Cut 4 (12-inch) squares of foil. Fold squares
    in half diagonally and lay each breast half to one side of
    diagonal crease.

4. Spoon 1 tablespoon tomatoes, 2 tablespoons chilies and ¼ cup
    corn on each chicken breast half. Loosely fold foil over chicken
    and seal edges.

5. Bake for 15 minutes and check chicken breasts for doneness. (Be
    careful when opening steaming packets.)

6. If chicken is still pink in center, reseal and bake about 5 minutes
    longer or until chicken is no longer pink.

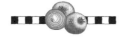

*Who doesn't love canned diced green chilies?
Keep several 4-ounce cans in your pantry for a
flavorful addition to recipes.*

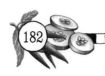

Slow Cooker Chicken Enchiladas

1 pound chicken breast tenders
1 (15 ounce) can red or green enchilada sauce
8 (6 inch) reduced-carbohydrate flour tortillas
1¼ cups shredded reduced-fat colby Jack
    cheese, divided

Nutrition Facts
Serving Size 1 enchilada
Servings Per Recipe 8
Amount Per Serving
Calories 221
Total Fat 9g
Cholesterol 48mg
Sodium 613mg
Total Carbohydrate 15g
Dietary Fiber 8g
Sugars 2g
Protein 20g

1. Rinse tenders and pat dry with paper towels.
    Brown in sprayed nonstick 10 to 12-inch
    skillet.

2. Transfer chicken to 4 to 5-quart slow cooker.
    Add enchilada sauce. Cook on LOW for
    3 to 4 hours or until chicken shreds easily.
    Drain and shred tenders. Reserve enchilada sauce.

3. Preheat oven to 350°.

4. Transfer enchilada sauce to sprayed nonstick 10 to 12-inch skillet
    on medium-high. Immediately dip tortillas in sauce, fill with
    2 tablespoons chicken and 2 tablespoons cheese.

5. Roll tightly and arrange in sprayed 9 x 13-inch baking dish.

6. Sprinkle with reserved cheese. Bake about 15 minutes or until
    cheese melts.

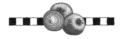

*The earliest enchiladas, in Mexico as in Texas,
were served in the street and usually nothing more
than a tortilla dipped in chile sauce, sometimes
sprinkled with cheese and chopped onions.*

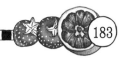
Hearty Chicken Burrito

1 tablespoon reduced-fat cream cheese
1 (8 inch) reduced-carbohydrate flour tortilla
2 tablespoons shredded cooked chicken breast
2 teaspoons chopped green onion

1. Preheat oven to 400°.

2. Spread cream cheese on tortilla and spoon chicken and onion on top.

3. Roll tortilla and place seam side down on sprayed foil-lined baking sheet. Spray rolled tortilla and heat 5 to 6 minutes.

Nutrition Facts		
Serving Size 1 burrito		
Servings Per Recipe 1		
Amount Per Serving		
Calories 172		
Total Fat 6g		
Cholesterol 23mg		
Sodium 397mg		
Total Carbohydrate 19g		
Dietary Fiber 18g		
Sugars 1g		
Protein 11g		

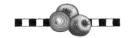

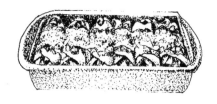

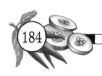

Dijon Grilled Chicken

½ cup bottled marinade for chicken, divided
3 tablespoons dijon-style mustard
2 tablespoons olive oil
4 (4 ounce) boneless skinless chicken breast
 halves (1 pound)

1. Mix marinade, dijon-style mustard and olive oil to make marinade.

2. Pour ¼ cup over chicken in plastic bag. Seal and refrigerate 1 to 3 hours. Refrigerate remaining marinade.

3. Remove chicken from plastic bag and discard used marinade. Grill or broil chicken and baste with reserved marinade, until no longer pink.

TIP: It's always best to discard the liquid used to marinate chicken. Use fresh marinade during the cooking process.

Nutrition Facts
Serving Size 1 chicken breast half
Servings Per Recipe 4
Amount Per Serving
Calories 216
Total Fat 10g
Cholesterol 76mg
Sodium 697mg
Total Carbohydrate 3g
Dietary Fiber 0g
Sugars 2g
Protein 25

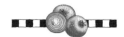

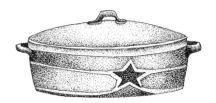

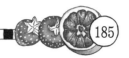
Crunchy Chicken Tenders

¾ pound chicken breast tenders
2 egg whites, beaten
½ cup corn flake crumbs
1 tablespoon olive oil

Nutrition Facts
Serving Size 3 chicken tenders
Servings Per Recipe 4
Amount Per Serving
Calories 175
Total Fat 6g
Cholesterol 55mg
Sodium 176mg
Total Carbohydrate 9g
Dietary Fiber 0g
Sugars 1g
Protein 21g

1. Rinse chicken tenders and pat dry with paper towels. Dip chicken tenders in egg white and coat with crumbs.

2. In nonstick 10 to 12-inch skillet, heat olive oil over medium-high heat. When oil is hot, add half the tenders. Cook about 3 to 4 minutes on each side.

3. If needed, reduce heat to medium. Cook remaining tenders.

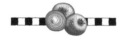

One suggested way to avoid flatulence from dried beans: Simmer beans in water for 30 minutes, drain off the water, and add fresh boiling water or other liquid. Continue cooking until done.

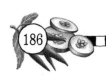

Teriyaki Chicken Tenders

1 pound chicken breast tenders
⅓ cup plus 2 teaspoons reduced-sodium teriyaki
    sauce, divided
¼ cup sliced green onion
1 (8 ounce) can pineapple tidbits with
    reduced-sugar juice

Nutrition Facts
Serving Size 2 chicken tenders
Servings Per Recipe 4
Amount Per Serving
Calories 178
Total Fat 3g
Cholesterol 73mg
Sodium 613mg
Total Carbohydrate 11g
Dietary Fiber 1g
Sugars 11g
Protein 25g

1. Seal tenders and ⅓ cup teriyaki sauce in plastic bag. Refrigerate 15 to 20 minutes. Remove and discard marinade.

2. Preheat sprayed nonstick wok or 10 to 12-inch skillet over high heat. Add about half chicken tenders. Cook and stir for 2 minutes or until chicken browns. Reduce heat as needed.

3. Remove first batch and repeat with remaining tenders. Remove second batch.

4. Drain juice from can of pineapple tidbits into small bowl.

5. Add green onions, pineapple, 1 tablespoon pineapple juice and 2 teaspoons remaining teriyaki sauce to skillet.

6. Cook and stir about 1 minute. Spoon over chicken tenders.

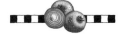

If a recipe calls for green onions, use both the white and green parts of the onion, unless otherwise specified.

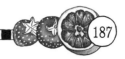
Chicken-Bell Pepper Medley

1 pound chicken breast tenders
1 tablespoon olive oil
3 assorted bell peppers (green, red or yellow),
    thinly sliced
1 medium onion, thinly sliced

Nutrition Facts
Serving Size ¼ chicken tenders and vegetables
Servings Per Recipe 4
Amount Per Serving
Calories 108
Total Fat 7g
Cholesterol 73mg
Sodium 136mg
Total Carbohydrate 8g
Dietary Fiber 2g
Sugars 5g
Protein 5g

1. Rinse chicken breast tenders and pat dry with paper towels.

2. Heat olive oil in nonstick 10 to 12-inch skillet over medium-high heat. Add tenders to the skillet and cook, turning once, until light brown. Remove from skillet.

3. Add peppers and onion to skillet. Cook and stir over medium heat until tender. Return chicken tenders to skillet and heat through.

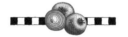

*An eggshell's color – either brown or white –
is determined by the breed of hen, not by taste or
nutritive value.*

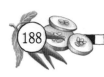

Breaded Chicken Cutlets

4 (4 ounce) skinless, boneless chicken breast
    halves (about 1 pound)
¼ cup panko (Japanese-style) breadcrumbs
¼ cup grated parmesan cheese
2 egg whites, beaten

Nutrition Facts		
Serving Size 2 cutlets		
Servings Per Recipe 5		
Amount Per Serving		
Calories 143		
Total Fat 4g		
Cholesterol 63mg		
Sodium 208mg		
Total Carbohydrate 3g		
Dietary Fiber 0g		
Sugars 0g		
Protein 23		

1. Slice chicken breast halves crosswise into 3 slices to make cutlets.

2. Mix breadcrumbs and cheese. Dip chicken cutlets in egg white and coat both sides with breadcrumbs.

3. In sprayed nonstick 10 to 12-inch skillet over medium heat, cook chicken 4 to 5 minutes on each side; spray as needed.

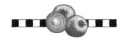

More statistical studies are finding that family meals play a significant role in childhood development. Children who eat with their families four or more nights per week are healthier, make better grades in school, score higher on aptitude tests and are less likely to have problems with drugs.

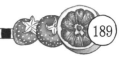
Chicken and Dumplings

7 tablespoons reduced-fat baking mix
¼ teaspoon dried thyme, crushed
2 (14 ounce) cans reduced-sodium fat-free
   chicken broth
1 (9¾ ounce) can fat-free chicken breast in
   water, drained

Nutrition Facts		
Serving Size ¾ cup		
Servings Per Recipe 6		
Amount Per Serving		
Calories 87		
Total Fat 1g		
Cholesterol 21mg		
Sodium 713mg		
Total Carbohydrate 8g		
Dietary Fiber 0g		
Sugars 1g		
Protein 10		

1. Stir together baking mix, 3 tablespoons water
   and thyme to make soft dough.

2. In 2 to 3-quart saucepan over medium-high
   heat, bring chicken broth to a boil.

3. Drop dumpling dough by tablespoonfuls onto boiling broth.
   Reduce heat to medium and cook uncovered 10 minutes.

4. Add chicken, cover and cook 10 minutes or until dumplings
   are cooked.

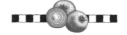

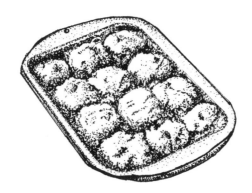

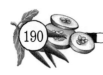

Creamy Spinach Chicken Rolls

4 (4 ounce) skinless, boneless chicken breast
    halves (1 pound)
½ cup finely chopped white mushrooms
½ (10 ounce) package frozen chopped spinach,
    squeezed dry
4 tablespoons reduced-fat cream cheese

Nutrition Facts
Serving Size 1 chicken roll
Servings Per Recipe 4
Amount Per Serving
Calories 182
Total Fat 6g
Cholesterol 84mg
Sodium 261mg
Total Carbohydrate 4g
Dietary Fiber 2g
Sugars 2g
Protein 28g

1. Lightly pound chicken between 2 large
   sheets of wax paper with rolling pin
   to flatten.

2. Cook and stir mushrooms for 2 to
   3 minutes in sprayed nonstick 10 to
   12-inch skillet over medium heat. Combine mushrooms,
   spinach and cream cheese.

3. Spoon 2 to 3 tablespoons on top of each chicken breast half. Roll
   and secure with cotton string or toothpicks and spray both sides.

4. Return skillet to medium-high heat and add chicken rolls.

5. Reduce heat to medium and cook rolls about 10 to 12 minutes
   or until chicken browns and is no longer pink. Spray skillet
   as needed.

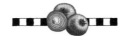

*Green vegetables such as spinach are a good
source of vitamin K, essential for blood clotting.*

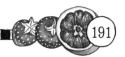
Company Chicken Rolls

4 (4 ounce) skinless, boneless chicken breast
  halves (1 pound)
½ (10 ounce) package frozen chopped
  spinach, thawed, squeezed dry
½ cup grated parmesan cheese
¼ cup soft "Lite Wheat Breadcrumbs," p. 226

Nutrition Facts	
Serving Size 1 chicken roll Amount Per Serving	
Amount Per Serving	
Calories 199	
Total Fat 7g	
Cholesterol 85mg	
Sodium 359mg	
Total Carbohydrate 3g	
Dietary Fiber 1g	
Sugars 0g	
Protein 30g	

1. Preheat oven to 425°.

2. Lightly pound chicken between 2 sheets of
    wax paper with rolling pin to flatten.

3. Combine spinach and parmesan cheese and
    spoon 2 to 3 tablespoons on chicken breast halves. Roll and secure
    with toothpicks.

4. Spray chicken and roll in breadcrumbs. Arrange chicken rolls
    seam-side down on sprayed foil-covered baking sheet. Spray tops
    of rolls lightly.

5. Bake until chicken is no longer pink and crust is golden, about
    25 minutes.

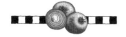

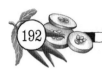

Lettuce Turkey Wraps

6 large lettuce leaves
6 thin slices deli smoked turkey breast
1 medium tomato, halved, sliced thinly
2 tablespoons fat-free ranch-style dressing

1. Top each lettuce leaf with turkey and tomato.

2. Drizzle with dressing and roll up tightly. Makes 6 lettuce wraps.

Nutrition Facts	
Serving Size 2 lettuce wraps	
Servings Per Recipe 3	
Amount Per Serving	
Calories 81	
Total Fat 1g	
Cholesterol 25mg	
Sodium 518mg	
Total Carbohydrate 5g	
Dietary Fiber 1g	
Sugars 4g	
Protein 14g	

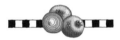

Whoever created lettuce wraps gave us a delicious sandwich option.

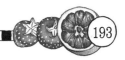

Turkey Sausage and Cabbage

1 large onion, chopped
2 medium carrots, sliced
6 cups coarsely shredded green cabbage
1 (14 ounce) package smoked turkey sausage,
    cut in bite-size pieces

1. Cook and stir onion and carrots until just
   tender in sprayed nonstick large, heavy pan
   over medium-high heat.

2. Reduce heat to medium and add cabbage
   and sausage. Cook, covered, for 15 to
   20 minutes, stirring frequently, until cabbage
   is tender.

Nutrition Facts	
Serving Size 1 cup	
Servings Per Recipe 6	
Amount Per Serving	
Calories 139	
Total Fat 6g	
Cholesterol 35mg	
Sodium 634mg	
Total Carbohydrate 12g	
Dietary Fiber 3g	
Sugars 6g	
Protein 11g	

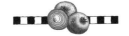

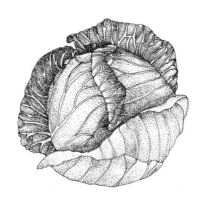

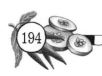

Turkey-Spaghetti Sauce

2 cloves garlic, minced
1 cup sliced small white mushrooms
1 pound ground turkey breast
3 cups "Homemade Marinara Sauce," p. 220

Nutrition Facts	
Serving Size ¾ cup	
Servings Per Recipe 6	
Amount Per Serving	
Calories 145	
Total Fat 1g	
Cholesterol 33mg	
Sodium 15mg	
Total Carbohydrate 17g	
Dietary Fiber 5g	
Sugars 10g	
Protein 14g	

1. Cook and stir garlic and mushrooms until tender in sprayed large, heavy pan on medium heat. Remove from pan.

2. Cook and stir turkey in same pan over medium heat until no longer pink.

3. Add garlic-mushroom mixture and marinara sauce and bring to a boil. Reduce heat and simmer for about 10 minutes.

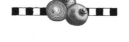

Here's an easy way to measure 4 ounces of long spaghetti. Make a circle about the size of a quarter with your thumb and index finger and fill it with pasta. Allow at least a quart of boiling water to cook each 4 ounces of pasta.

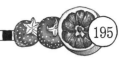

Turkey Cutlets with Fruit Sauce

4 medium turkey breast cutlets
1 medium Granny Smith apple, cored, finely
    chopped
2 tablespoons sweetened dried cranberries
2 teaspoons finely grated orange peel
    plus 2 tablespoons orange juice

Nutrition Facts
Serving Size 1 cutlet with sauce
Servings Per Recipe 4
Amount Per Serving
Calories 168
Total Fat 1g
Cholesterol 70mg
Sodium 56mg
Total Carbohydrate 12g
Dietary Fiber 30g
Sugars 9g
Protein 28g

1. Cook cutlets about 3 minutes on each side or until no longer pink in sprayed nonstick 10 to 12-inch skillet over medium heat. Remove from skillet.

2. Add apple, cranberries, orange peel and juice to skillet. Over medium heat, cook and stir about 4 minutes. Spoon over cutlets.

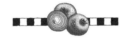

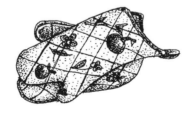

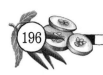

Sausage Cheese-Stuffed Poblanos

4 medium poblano chilies
½ pound hot Italian turkey sausage, casings
    removed
1 cup reduced-fat cottage cheese, drained
½ cup reduced-fat shredded mozzarella
    cheese

Nutrition Facts	
Serving Size 1 stuffed chile	
Servings Per Recipe 4	
Amount Per Serving	
Calories 149	
Total Fat 5g	
Cholesterol 27mg	
Sodium 628mg	
Total Carbohydrate 7g	
Dietary Fiber 1g	
Sugars 4g	
Protein 20g	

1. Preheat broiler.

2. Split poblano chilies with sharp knife and remove seeds, but leave stems on. Rinse and pat dry on paper towels.

3. On foil-covered baking sheet, 4 to 5 inches from heat, broil chilies on all sides until skin chars.

4. Remove and seal in plastic bag. When cool, carefully peel skin away.

5. Preheat oven to 350°.

6. Brown sausage in 10 to 12-inch skillet on medium-high heat. Combine sausage with cottage cheese.

7. Spoon sausage mixture into chilies and sprinkle each with 2 tablespoons mozzarella cheese. Bake for 15 minutes or until cheese melts.

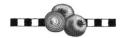

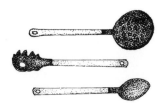

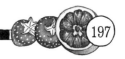

Canadian Bacon Pizzas

2 multi-grain sandwich thins or flats, halved
¼ cup pizza sauce
2 (1 ounce) slices Canadian bacon, chopped
¼ cup shredded reduced-fat mozzarella cheese

1. Lightly toast sandwich thin halves in oven. Remove and spread 2 tablespoons pizza sauce on each half. Sprinkle bacon and cheese on top.

2. Set oven on broil, add sandwich thin halves and broil just until cheese melts.

Nutrition Facts
Serving Size 1 pizza
Servings Per Recipe 4
Amount Per Serving
Calories 145
Total Fat 5g
Cholesterol 25mg
Sodium 825mg
Total Carbohydrate 13g
Dietary Fiber 3g
Sugars 1g
Protein 13g

TIP: If you have a toaster oven, this is a great recipe for it. You don't have to heat up the kitchen and you get excellent results with a toaster oven.

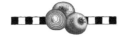

Strange as it may seem, Americans are the only ones on the planet to use the term, "Canadian bacon." Even Canadians use just the term "bacon." Well, it is reported that Canadian bacon is made from pigs either raised or slaughtered in Canada.

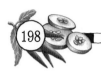

Dijon Pork Chops

½ cup plain panko (Japanese-style)
    breadcrumbs
1 tablespoon chopped parsley
4 (4 ounce) boneless pork chops, trimmed
4 teaspoons dijon-style mustard

Nutrition Facts
Serving Size 1 pork chop
Servings Per Recipe 4
Amount Per Serving
Calories 162
Total Fat 4g
Cholesterol 64mg
Sodium 182mg
Total Carbohydrate 6g
Dietary Fiber 0g
Sugars 1g
Protein 22g

1. Preheat oven to 350°.

2. Combine bread crumbs and parsley. Spread one side of pork chops with ½ teaspoon mustard and coat in crumbs. Repeat with other side.

3. Bake pork chops on sprayed foil-covered baking sheet about 30 minutes or until pork is tender and no longer pink.

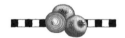

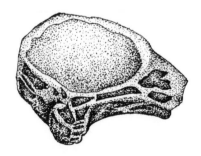

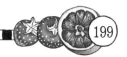
Slow Cooked Barbecued Pork Chops

4 (¾-inch) thick boneless pork chops, trimmed
¾ cup "Low-Carb Barbecue Sauce," p. 223

1. In sprayed nonstick 10 to 12-inch skillet on medium-high heat, brown pork chops on both sides. Transfer to 4 to 5-quart slow cooker.

2. Pour barbecue sauce over pork chops. Cover and cook on LOW for 4 to 6 hours or until pork is very tender.

Nutrition Facts	
Serving Size 1 pork chop	
Servings Per Recipe 4	
Amount Per Serving	
Calories 210	
Total Fat 4g	
Cholesterol 74mg	
Sodium 621mg	
Total Carbohydrate 8g	
Dietary Fiber 0g	
Sugars 8g	
Protein 34g	

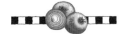

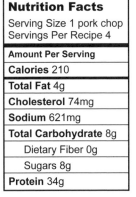

If you are trying to lose weight, one tip is to go meatless at least twice each week. Instead of meat, try dried peas and beans, grains, vegetables and fruits, which also give you a fiber boost.

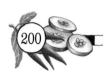

All-Day Pork Loin Roast and Vegetables

1 (1 pound) package frozen stew vegetables
1 (2 pound) boneless pork loin roast, cut in
    1-inch pieces
1 (14 ounce) can no-salt diced tomatoes
½ teaspoon dried thyme, crushed

Nutrition Facts
Serving Size ¾ cup pork and vegetables
Servings Per Recipe 8
Amount Per Serving
Calories 161
Total Fat 5g
Cholesterol 55mg
Sodium 217mg
Total Carbohydrate 28g
Dietary Fiber 1g
Sugars 2g
Protein 25g

1. Pour frozen stew vegetables in 4 to 5-quart slow cooker.

2. Brown pork in sprayed nonstick 10 to 12-inch skillet over medium-high heat and transfer to slow cooker.

3. Add tomatoes and thyme and cook on LOW for 6 to 8 hours or until pork is very tender.

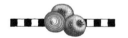

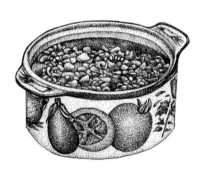

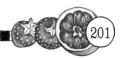
Surprise Pulled Pork

1 (2 pound) pork tenderloin, trimmed
1 cup diet root beer
1¼ cups "Low-Carb Barbecue Sauce," p. 223

Nutrition Facts		
Serving size ¾ cup pork Servings Per Recipe 8		
Amount Per Serving		
Calories 146		
Total Fat 2g		
Cholesterol 74mg		
Sodium 425mg		
Total Carbohydrate 5g		
Dietary Fiber 0g		
Sugars 10g		
Protein 24g		

1. Rinse tenderloin and pat dry with paper towels. In sprayed nonstick 10 to 12-inch skillet, brown tenderloin on all sides.

2. Transfer to 4 to 5-quart slow cooker. Pour root beer in bottom and barbecue sauce on top of pork.

3. Cook on LOW for 4 to 6 hours or until pork shreds easily.

On the ingredients list on a canned or packaged food, ingredients are listed in order by weight (high to low), so the first ingredients make up most of the food.

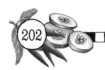

Home-Style Pork Meatballs

¼ cup liquid egg substitute
1 slice light-style wheat bread, torn in
    small pieces
¾ pound lean ground pork
2 (4g) packets sodium-free beef broth
    and seasoning

Nutrition Facts	
Serving Size 2 meatballs	
Servings Per Recipe 5	
Amount Per Serving	
Calories 166	
Total Fat 11g	
Cholesterol 46mg	
Sodium 86mg	
Total Carbohydrate 3g	
Dietary Fiber 0g	
Sugars 1g	
Protein 14g	

1. Mix egg, bread and pork. Shape into
    10 (2-inch) balls.

2. Bring 2 cups water to a boil in large, heavy
    pan. Stir in broth packets. Carefully drop
    meatballs in broth with tongs. Reduce heat
    and cover.

3. Simmer meatballs for 30 minutes or until no longer pink.

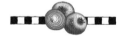

Quick and easy estimates of portion sizes:

> *3 ounces meat is about the size of a deck
>   of cards*
>
> *1 cup cooked vegetables is about the size of
>   your fist*
>
> *1 small fruit is about the size of a tennis ball*
>
> *½ cup ice cream is about the size of
>   a racquetball*

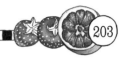
Pork Chops with Apricot Sauce

4 (4 ounce) boneless pork chops, trimmed
½ teaspoon poultry seasoning
⅔ cup "Apricot Sauce for Pork," p. 224
½ cup sliced green onion

1. Sprinkle poultry seasoning on pork chops and brown in sprayed nonstick 10 to 12-inch skillet over medium-high heat.

2. Add apricot sauce to skillet and bring to a boil. Reduce heat, cover, and simmer for 20 minutes or until pork is no longer pink. Garnish with green onions.

Nutrition Facts	
Serving Size 1 pork chop with sauce	
Servings per Recipe 4	
Amount Per Serving	
Calories 170	
Total Fat 4g	
Cholesterol 75mg	
Sodium 59mg	
Total Carbohydrate 7g	
Dietary Fiber 0g	
Sugars 9g	
Protein 26g	

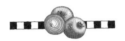

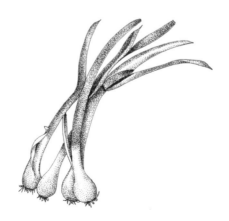

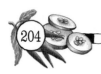

Hawaiian Ham Steak

1 cup coarsely chopped yellow bell pepper
1 (8 ounce) package ham steaks
½ cup reduced-sugar pineapple tidbits, drained
¾ cup "Hawaiian Ham Sauce," p. 222

Nutrition Facts	
Serving Size ¼ portion	
Servings Per Recipe 4	
Amount Per Serving	
Calories 108	
Total Fat 1g	
Cholesterol 23mg	
Sodium 764mg	
Total Carbohydrate 14g	
Dietary Fiber 0g	
Sugars 9g	
Protein 11g	

1. Cook and stir bell pepper for about 4 to
   5 minutes or until lightly browned in sprayed
   nonstick 10 to 12-inch skillet over medium
   heat. Remove bell pepper from skillet.

2. Cut ham steaks in half. In same skillet over
   medium heat, lightly brown ham. Remove
   from skillet and keep warm.

3. Add bell pepper, pineapple and sauce to skillet. Bring to a boil,
   reduce heat and simmer until heats through. Pour over ham.

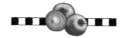

One pound of body fat is equal to 3,500 calories.

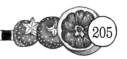

Seaside Fish Tacos

2 medium (8 ounce) tilapia fillets or other
    firm-flesh fish fillets
4 (6-inch) flour tortillas
1 cup shredded red cabbage
"Fish Taco Sauce," p. 220

Nutrition Facts	
Serving Size 1 taco	
Servings Per Recipe 4	
Amount Per Serving	
Calories 154	
Total Fat 4g	
Cholesterol 26mg	
Sodium 240mg	
Total Carbohydrate 17g	
Dietary Fiber 1g	
Sugars 2g	
Protein 13g	

1. On sprayed, foil-lined broiler pan, broil fillets about 5 inches from heat until fish flakes. Cut fillets in half lengthwise.

2. On each tortilla, place half fillet, ¼ cup shredded cabbage and 2 tablespoons sauce. Roll or fold tortilla.

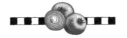

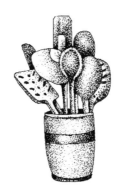

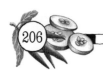

Creole Broiled Catfish

4 (4 ounce) catfish fillets
2 teaspoons Creole seasoning
1 lemon, cut in wedges

Nutrition Facts	
Serving Size 1 fillet	
Servings Per Recipe 4	
Amount Per Serving	
Calories 152	
Total Fat 9g	
Cholesterol 53mg	
Sodium 406mg	
Total Carbohydrate 0g	
Dietary Fiber 0g	
Sugars 0g	
Protein 18g	

1. Preheat broiler.

2. Rinse fillets and pat dry with paper towels. Spray both sides and sprinkle with seasoning.

3. Place fillets on sprayed broiler pan about 5 inches from heat. Broil each side for about 6 minutes or until fish is crispy and flakes easily with fork. Serve with lemon wedges.

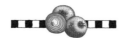

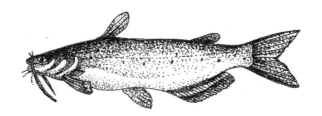

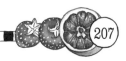

Grilled Halibut Fillets

½ cup fresh lemon juice
2 medium jalapeño chilies, seeded, finely
    chopped*
4 (6 ounce) frozen halibut fillets
¼ cup coarsely chopped cilantro

Nutrition Facts
Serving Size 1 fillet
Servings Per Recipe 4
Amount Per Serving
Calories 196
Total Fat 4g
Cholesterol 55mg
Sodium 93mg
Total Carbohydrate 3g
Dietary Fiber 0g
Sugars 1g
Protein 36g

1. Stir together lemon juice and chilies.

2. Seal fish fillets and lemon juice mixture in plastic bag. Refrigerate 30 minutes, turning once. Remove halibut and reserve marinade.

3. On charcoal or gas grill, place fish directly on rack and grill 3 to 5 minutes. Turn once and grill additional 2 to 3 minutes and brush with marinade. Sprinkle with cilantro.

TIP: Wear rubber gloves when removing seeds from jalapeños.

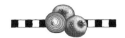

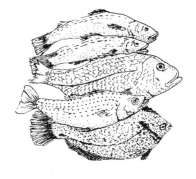

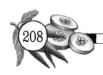

Marinated Baked Salmon

1 (16 ounce) package frozen salmon fillets
3 tablespoons reduced-sodium soy sauce
2 tablespoons lemon juice
Chopped parsley

1. Thaw salmon fillets according to package instructions and pat dry with paper towels. Seal fillets, soy sauce and lemon juice in plastic bag and refrigerate 1 hour.

2. Preheat oven to 375°.

3. Drain fillets and center each on sprayed foil rectangle. Fold foil over fillets, place on baking sheet and bake for 30 minutes or until salmon flakes easily. Garnish with parsley.

Nutrition Facts	
Serving Size 4 ounce fillet	
Servings Per Recipe 4	
Amount Per Serving	
Calories 110	
Total Fat 3g	
Cholesterol 45mg	
Sodium 701mg	
Total Carbohydrate 1g	
Dietary Fiber 0g	
Sugars 0g	
Protein 20g	

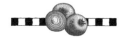

Salmon is a major source of omega-3 fats, found to reduce risks of heart disease and stroke. The American Heart Association recommends two servings of fish a week, with an emphasis on fatty fish such as salmon, herring and mackerel.

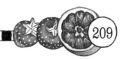
Skillet Salmon Patties

1 (12 ounce) can salmon, drained, flaked
⅓ cup finely chopped onion
¼ cup liquid egg substitute
¾ cup (21) crushed multi-grain saltine crackers, divided

Nutrition Facts		
Serving Size 1 patty		
Servings Per Recipe 6		
Amount Per Serving		
Calories 129		
Total Fat 4g		
Cholesterol 31mg		
Sodium 453mg		
Total Carbohydrate 8g		
Dietary Fiber 0g		
Sugars 1g		
Protein 12g		

1. Mix salmon, onion, egg substitute and ¼ cup crumbs.

2. Measure ⅓ cup salmon mixture for each patty. Form into 6 patties and coat with remaining crumbs.

3. Preheat sprayed nonstick 10 to 12-inch skillet over medium-high heat. Cook each side of patty for about 3 minutes.

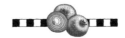

Most people don't eat enough fiber. Sometimes it's easier to grab juice instead of whole fruit, or high-calorie snacks instead of cutting fresh vegetables. Fiber or roughage, as it is called, offers many health benefits. It's worth any small amount of effort!

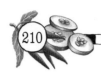

Super Supper Salmon Loaf

2 slices light-style wheat bread, torn in
　　small pieces
¼ cup finely chopped onion
2 egg whites, beaten
1 (15 ounce) can salmon, drained, flaked

Nutrition Facts	
Serving Size 1-inch slice	
Servings Per Recipe 8	
Amount Per Serving	
Calories 95	
Total Fat 5g	
Cholesterol 35mg	
Sodium 270mg	
Total Carbohydrate 3g	
Dietary Fiber 1g	
Sugars 0g	
Protein 12g	

1. Preheat oven to 350°.

2. Stir together bread, onion, egg whites and
   2 tablespoons water. Let stand for 5 minutes.
   Add salmon and mix thoroughly.

3. Spread salmon mixture into sprayed
   5 x 9-inch loaf pan. Bake 50 to 55 minutes or until lightly
   browned. Let stand about 10 minutes before cutting.

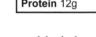

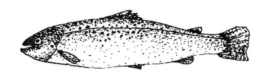

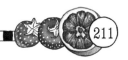

Baked Salmon Special

1 (1 pound) package frozen salmon fillets
½ (10 ounce) package frozen chopped spinach, thawed, squeezed dry
2 tablespoons onion-chive flavored cream cheese, softened
4 teaspoons lemon juice

Nutrition Facts	
Serving Size 4 ounces	
Servings Per Recipe 4	
Amount Per Serving	
Calories 141	
Total Fat 5g	
Cholesterol 51mg	
Sodium 350mg	
Total Carbohydrate 4g	
Dietary Fiber 2g	
Sugars 1g	
Protein 22g	

1. Thaw salmon fillets according to package instructions. Drain and pat dry with paper towels.

2. Preheat oven to 375°.

3. Mix spinach and cream cheese. Place each salmon fillet on sprayed foil rectangle.

4. Spread ¼ cup spinach mixture on top of fillets. Fold and seal foil over fillets.

5. Bake 30 minutes or until salmon flakes easily. Sprinkle each fillet with 1 teaspoon lemon juice.

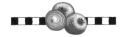

Most recently, mercury poisoning from fish has been a concern; however, fish for consumption in the U.S. meet safety standards for mercury and other contaminants. Fortunately, salmon, a rich source of omega-3 fats, is relatively low in mercury.

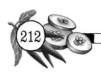

Tuna Melt Muffin

2 (2½ ounce) pouches solid white albacore
    tuna in water, drained
2 tablespoons reduced-fat mayonnaise
2 whole wheat English muffins, split
4 slices fat-free sharp cheddar cheese

1. Flake tuna and mix with mayonnaise.
   Spread 2 tablespoons on muffin half and top
   with cheese.

2. In toaster oven, broil until cheese melts and
   muffin browns.

Nutrition Facts	
Serving Size 1 muffin half	
Servings Per Recipe 4	
Amount Per Serving	
Calories 182	
Total Fat 6g	
Cholesterol 24mg	
Sodium 563mg	
Total Carbohydrate 15g	
Dietary Fiber 3g	
Sugars 3g	
Protein 19g	

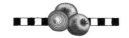

Should people with diabetes eat special diabetic foods? Diabetic and "dietetic" foods generally offer no special benefit. Most of them are usually more expensive than wisely-chosen healthy foods and will still raise blood glucose levels.

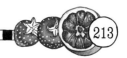

Shrimp Florentine

2 (10 ounce) bags washed fresh spinach
1 tablespoon cornstarch
2 pounds frozen cooked medium shrimp, peeled, veined, thawed, drained
½ teaspoon lemon pepper seasoning

Nutrition Facts	
Service Size 1 cup	
Servings Per Recipe 8	
Amount Per Serving	
Calories 140	
Total Fat 2g	
Cholesterol 172mg	
Sodium 313mg	
Total Carbohydrate 4g	
Dietary Fiber 1g	
Sugars 0g	
Protein 25g	

1. In sprayed nonstick 10 to 12-inch skillet over medium heat, cook spinach for 3 to 5 minutes or until it is limp. Add a small amount of water if needed.

2. Mix cornstarch with 1 tablespoon water and stir to dissolve. Add cornstarch to spinach, bring to a boil, and stir until it thickens.

3. Reduce heat to low, add shrimp and sprinkle with seasoning. Cook just until heated through.

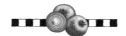

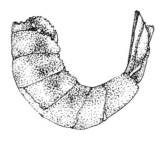

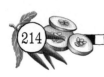

Creole Shrimp

1 (12 ounce) package frozen chopped onion,
     bell peppers, celery and parsley blend
2 (8 ounce) cans no-salt tomato sauce
½ teaspoon Creole seasoning
¾ pound fresh medium shrimp, shelled, tails
     removed, veined

Nutrition Facts		
Serving Size 1 cup		
Servings Per Recipe 4		
Amount Per Serving		
Calories 171		
Total Fat 1g		
Cholesterol 129mg		
Sodium 211mg		
Total Carbohydrate 17g		
Dietary Fiber 4g		
Sugars 10g		
Protein 19g		

1. In sprayed nonstick 10 to 12-inch skillet
   over medium-high heat, cook and stir onion-
   mixture until tender.

2. Add tomato sauce, ½ cup water and
   seasoning. Bring to a boil, reduce heat and
   simmer about 5 minutes.

3. Add shrimp and cook just until shrimp turns pink.

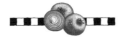

*Shellfish, such as shrimp, are a significant source
of vitamin B$_{12}$ as are animal-based foods. After
years of consuming only plant products, a person
might develop a deficiency of B$_{12}$, so important for
the body's metabolism and maintenance of nerve cells.*

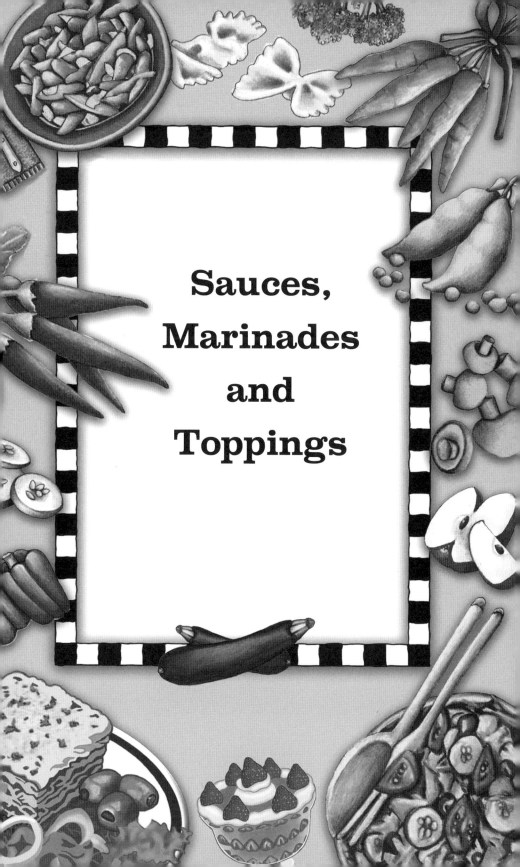

Sauces,
Marinades
and
Toppings

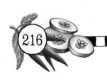

Sauces, Marinades and Toppings Contents

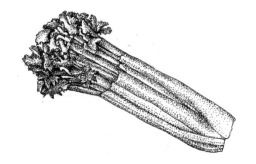

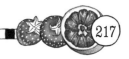
Sally's Seasoning Blend

2 cloves garlic, minced
1⅓ cups finely chopped onion
1 cup chopped red or green bell pepper
1 cup chopped celery

1. In sprayed nonstick 10 to 12-inch skillet, cook and stir all vegetables until tender.

2. Ready for use in recipes calling for frozen chopped onions, peppers, celery and parsley blend. Makes 3 cups.

TIP: If you need a timesaver, you can buy a similar seasoning blending in the frozen food section of the grocery store or make this recipe and freeze it.

Nutrition Facts	
Serving Size ½ cup	
Servings Per Recipe 6	
Amount Per Serving	
Calories 43	
Total Fat 0g	
Cholesterol 0mg	
Sodium 16mg	
Total Carbohydrate 6g	
Dietary Fiber 1g	
Sugars 3g	
Protein 1g	

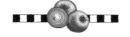

Remove garlic odor from your hands by rubbing them with lemon, then with salt. Rinse, then wash with soap and warm water.

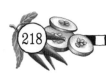

Simple Stir-Fry Sauce

2 tablespoons reduced-sodium soy sauce
1 teaspoon sesame oil
½ teaspoon peeled, minced ginger root
¼ - ½ teaspoon crushed red pepper

1. Whisk ingredients together. Makes
   3 tablespoons.

Nutrition Facts	
Serving Size 2 teaspoons	
Servings Per Recipe 6	
Amount Per Serving	
Calories 11	
Total Fat 1g	
Cholesterol 0mg	
Sodium 193mg	
Total Carbohydrate 0g	
Dietary Fiber 0g	
Sugars 0g	
Protein 0g	

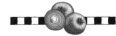

Seafood Cocktail Sauce

¼ cup reduced-sugar ketchup
¼ cup reduced-fat mayonnaise
2 tablespoons finely chopped onion
1 tablespoon lemon juice

1. Stir ingredients together in small bowl and
   refrigerate. Makes ¾ cup.

Nutrition Facts	
Serving Size 2 tablespoons	
Servings Per Recipe 6	
Amount Per Serving	
Calories 29	
Total Fat 2g	
Cholesterol 3mg	
Sodium 214mg	
Total Carbohydrate 2g	
Dietary Fiber 0g	
Sugars 0g	
Protein 0g	

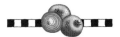

Weight Management: Limit high fat foods.

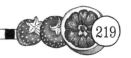
Easy Pizza Sauce

1 (8 ounce) can no-salt-added tomato sauce
1 (6 ounce) can no-salt-added tomato paste
1 teaspoon dried basil, crushed

1. In 1½ to 2-quart saucepan, cook and stir
   ingredients on medium heat for about
   3 minutes. Makes 1½ cups.

Nutrition Facts	
Serving Size 1 tablespoon	
Servings Per Recipe 24	
Amount Per Serving	
Calories 11	
Total Fat 0g	
Cholesterol 0mg	
Sodium 5mg	
Total Carbohydrate 2g	
Dietary Fiber 1g	
Sugars 1g	
Protein 0g	

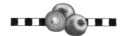

The innovation that gave us the flatbread we call pizza was the use of tomato as a topping. During the 18th century in Naples, Italy, poor people added tomato to yeast-rising flatbread and pizza was born!

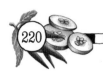

Fish Taco Sauce

½ cup reduced-fat mayonnaise
¼ cup reduced-fat sour cream
1 - 2 teaspoons Louisiana hot sauce
2 tablespoons lemon juice

1. Whisk ingredients and refrigerate. Makes ¾ cup.

Nutrition Facts
Serving Size 1 tablespoon
Servings Per Recipe 12
Amount Per Serving
Calories 37
Total Fat 3g
Cholesterol 7mg
Sodium 98mg
Total Carbohydrate 2g
Dietary Fiber 0g
Sugars 1g
Protein 1g

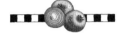

Homemade Marinara Sauce

1 (12 ounce) package frozen chopped onions, celery, peppers and parsley blend, thawed
2 cloves garlic, minced
2½ cups no-salt tomato sauce
2 teaspoons Italian herb seasoning, crushed

1. In sprayed large, heavy pan over medium heat, cook and stir onion mixture and garlic until tender. Add tomato sauce and herbs and bring to a boil.

2. Reduce heat and simmer, covered, for 10 to 15 minutes. Makes 3 cups.

Nutrition Facts
Serving Size ½ cup
Servings Per Recipe 6
Amount Per Serving
Calories 62
Total Fat 0g
Cholesterol 0mg
Sodium 12mg
Total Carbohydrate 13g
Dietary Fiber 4g
Sugars 7g
Protein 1g

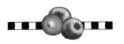

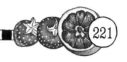

Speedy Mushroom Pasta Sauce

3 cups frozen chopped onion, celery, bell
    pepper and parsley blend
1½ cups sliced small fresh white mushrooms
1 (14 ounce) can diced tomatoes with basil,
    garlic and oregano
1 (6 ounce) can no-salt tomato paste

Nutrition Facts	
Serving Size ½ cup	
Servings Per Recipe 6	
Amount Per Serving	
Calories 75	
Total Fat 0g	
Cholesterol 0g	
Sodium 63mg	
Total Carbohydrate 15g	
Dietary Fiber 2g	
Sugars 10g	
Protein 3g	

1. In sprayed large, heavy pan over medium heat, cook and stir onion mixture about 5 minutes.

2. Stir in mushrooms and cook just until vegetables become tender. Spray as needed.

3. Whisk tomato paste and 2 cups water until smooth. Add tomato paste mixture and tomatoes to pan with vegetables.

4. Cook and stir over medium heat. Add small amount water as needed, until sauce thickens and is fragrant. Makes 3 cups.

TIP: Want a speedy way to slice mushrooms? Use an egg slicer!

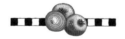

"Empty calories" is a term used to describe foods that have calories but no nutrients, such as sodas.

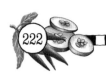

Veggie Pasta Sauce

3 cups frozen chopped onion, celery, bell
    peppers and parsley blend
½ cup chopped carrots
1 (14 ounce) can diced tomatoes with basil,
    garlic and oregano
1 (6 ounce) can no-salt tomato paste

Nutrition Facts	
Serving Size ½ cup	
Servings Per Recipe 6	
Amount Per Serving	
Calories 75	
Total Fat 0g	
Cholesterol 0mg	
Sodium 70mg	
Total Carbohydrate 15g	
Dietary Fiber 2g	
Sugars 10g	
Protein 3g	

1. In sprayed large, heavy pan over medium heat, cook and stir onion mixture and carrots about 15-20 minutes or until tender.

2. Stir tomato paste into 2 cups water until smooth. Add tomato paste mixture and tomatoes to pan with vegetables.

3. Cook and stir over medium heat and add water as needed until sauce thickens and is fragrant. Makes 3 cups.

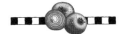

Hawaiian Ham Sauce

½ cup pineapple juice
1 tablespoon packed brown sugar
1 tablespoon corn starch
1 tablespoon cider vinegar

Nutrition Facts	
Serving Size 1 tablespoon	
Servings Per Recipe 16	
Amount Per Serving	
Calories 13	
Total Fat 0g	
Cholesterol 0mg	
Sodium 1mg	
Total Carbohydrate 3g	
Dietary Fiber 0g	
Sugars 2g	
Protein 0g	

1. Stir all ingredients and ¼ cup water together in 1½ to 2-quart saucepan. Cook and stir on medium heat until mixture thickens. Makes 1 cup.

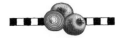

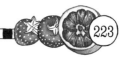

Low-Carb Barbecue Sauce

½ cup reduced-sugar ketchup
¼ cup cider vinegar
1 tablespoon molasses
1 teaspoon dry barbecue seasoning mix

1. Whisk all ingredients together. Store in refrigerator. Makes ¾ cup.

Nutrition Facts	
Serving Size 1 tablespoon Servings Per Recipe 12	
Amount Per Serving	
Calories 8	
Total Fat 0g	
Cholesterol 0mg	
Sodium 127mg	
Total Carbohydrate 2g	
Dietary Fiber 0g	
Sugars 4g	
Protein 0g	

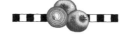

Over the years, the spelling of the tomato-based condiment as "ketchup" or "catsup" has been in question. Actually, "catsup" was the earlier spelling and is still used in southern U.S. and Mexico. However, "ketchup" is now the accepted spelling for the popular condiment throughout the world.

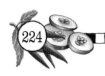

Apricot Sauce for Pork

1 (15 ounce) can apricot halves in juice
1 tablespoon cornstarch
¼ cup sugar-free apricot preserves
2 tablespoons white wine vinegar

Nutrition Facts
Serving Size ¼ cup
Servings Per Recipe 8
Amount Per Serving
Calories 35
Total Fat 0g
Cholesterol 0mg
Sodium 4mg
Total Carbohydrate 10g
Dietary Fiber 0g
Sugars 7g
Protein 0g

1. Drain apricot halves and reserve ⅔ cup juice. Slice apricot halves.

2. In 1½ to 2 quart saucepan, stir juice, cornstarch and vinegar together until cornstarch dissolves.

3. Bring to a boil, cook and stir continuously over medium heat until sauce thickens. Stir in preserves and apricots. Makes about 2 cups.

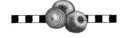

Apricots have been grown in China for some 4,000 years. In the U.S., California produces 90 percent of apricots consumed by Americans today.

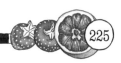
Beef Fajita Marinade

1 tablespoon lime juice
3 garlic cloves, peeled, halved
2 tablespoons olive oil
⅛ teaspoon ground cumin

1. Mix all ingredients. Makes about 3 tablespoons.

2. Seal one pound beef and marinade in large plastic bag. Marinate for 1 to 4 hours in refrigerator. Drain before use.

Nutrition Facts	
Serving Size 2 teaspoons Servings Per Recipe 10	
Amount Per Serving	
Calories 7	
Total Fat 0g	
Cholesterol 0mg	
Sodium 1mg	
Total Carbohydrate 2g	
Dietary Fiber 0g	
Sugars 0g	
Protein 0g	

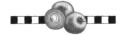

Ginger-Orange Marinade

1 teaspoon finely grated orange peel
    and 3 tablespoons juice
1 tablespoon white wine vinegar
1 teaspoon olive oil
1 teaspoon grated ginger

1. Whisk orange peel and juice with vinegar, oil and ginger. Makes ¼ cup.

TIP: Fresh ginger is more easily grated if stored in the freezer for a few hours.

Nutrition Facts	
Serving Size 1½ teaspoons Servings Per Recipe 8	
Amount Per Serving	
Calories 9	
Total Fat 1g	
Cholesterol 0mg	
Sodium 0g	
Total Carbohydrate 1g	
Dietary Fiber 0g	
Sugars 0g	
Protein 0g	

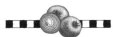

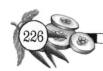

Lite Wheat Breadcrumbs

4 slices light-style wheat bread

1. Preheat oven to 250°.

2. Process one slice bread at a time in blender to make ½ cup soft fine crumbs.

3. Spread crumbs from 4 slices bread on baking sheet.

4. Bake 40 minutes and stir after 20 minutes. Makes about 1 cup toasted fine breadcrumbs.

Nutrition Facts
Serving Size 2 tablespoons
Servings Per Recipe 8
Amount Per Serving
Calories 20
Total Fat 0g
Cholesterol 0mg
Sodium 40mg
Total Carbohydrate 5g
Dietary Fiber 1g
Sugars 0g
Protein 1g

TIP: Calorie Fact: One slice of reduced-calorie bread has 20 fewer calories on average than one slice of regular bread.

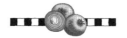

A food may be high in sugar if its ingredients list begins with or includes: sugar, sucrose, fructose, maltose, lactose, honey, syrup, corn syrup, high-fructose corn syrup, molasses or fruit juice concentrate.

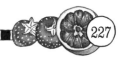
Ricotta Cream Topping

Make a delicious dessert by drizzling this creamy topping over fresh strawberries or blueberries.

1 cup part-skim ricotta cheese
2 tablespoons honey
1 tablespoon finely grated lemon peel
2 drops almond extract

1. Mix all ingredients until smooth in a blender on medium speed. Refrigerate 1 hour. Makes about 1¼ cups.

Nutrition Facts	
Serving Size ¼ cup	
Servings Per Recipe 4	
Amount Per Serving	
Calories 118	
Total Fat 5g	
Cholesterol 19mg	
Sodium 78mg	
Total Carbohydrate 12g	
Dietary Fiber 0g	
Sugars 9g	
Protein 7g	

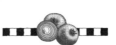

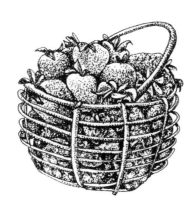

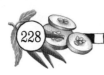

Crispy Fruit Topping

⅔ cup quick-cooking oatmeal
1 tablespoons packed brown sugar
    substitute blend
1 tablespoon flour
2 tablespoons melted butter

1. Mix oatmeal, brown sugar and flour. Stir in melted butter until ingredients are moist. Use with 2 to 3 cups fruit.

Nutrition Facts	
Serving Size 2 tablespoons Servings Per Recipe 8	
Amount Per Serving	
Calories 58	
Total Fat 3g	
Cholesterol 8mg	
Sodium 0mg	
Total Carbohydrate 6g	
Dietary Fiber 1g	
Sugars 1g	
Protein 1g	

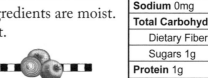

Liquid high-fructose corn syrup, made from corn starch in which some of the glucose has been converted to fructose, is the predominant sweetener in beverages and processed foods. Compared to sucrose (sugar), high-fructose corn syrup is less expensive, easier to use and is more stable.

Desserts

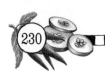

Desserts Contents

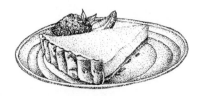

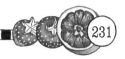

Apple Brown Betty

3 medium apples, cored, peeled, thinly sliced
¼ cup packed brown sugar-sugar substitute
    blend
2 tablespoons butter, chopped, divided
1½ cups soft light-style wheat breadcrumbs,
    divided

Nutrition Facts	
Serving Size ½ cup	
Servings Per Recipe 6	
Amount per Serving	
Calories 109	
Total Fat 4g	
Cholesterol 0mg	
Sodium 33mg	
Total Carbohydrate 17g	
Dietary Fiber 2g	
Sugars 11g	
Protein 1g	

1. Preheat oven to 350°.

2. Add apples and enough water to cover to boil in medium saucepan.

3. Reduce heat and simmer until apples are just tender. Drain apples and combine with brown sugar.

4. Place apples and ¼ cup water in 9 x 9-inch baking dish. Sprinkle apples with breadcrumbs and dot with butter.

5. Bake uncovered for 15 minutes or until breadcrumbs brown.

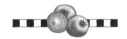

Small cakes, low-fat cookies or mini candy bars may occasionally be eaten as a snack, but check the food label for total number of carbohydrates per serving. Be sure the snack will fit into your food plan.

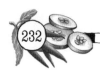

Pear Crisp

1 (14½ ounce) can no-sugar-added sliced pears,
    drained
½ teaspoon ground cinnamon
¼ cup chopped pecans
1 cup "Crispy Fruit Topping," p. 228

Nutrition Facts
Serving Size ½ cup
Servings Per Recipe 10
Amount Per Serving
Calories 39
Total Fat 2g
Cholesterol 1mg
Sodium 4mg
Total Carbohydrate 5g
Dietary Fiber 1g
Sugars 3g
Protein 0g

1. Preheat oven to 375°.

2. Arrange pears in 2-quart baking dish.
   Sprinkle with spice and pecans.

3. Spoon topping over pears and bake for
   15 minutes or until topping browns.

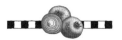

*Brown sugar has 17 calories per teaspoon as
compared to 13 calories per teaspoon of sugar.
Brown sugar is made by adding molasses to
refined sugar.*

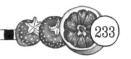
Creamy Fresh Fruit Pie

1 (8 ounce) carton fat-free sour cream
Sugar substitute equal to 2 tablespoons sugar
1 (9 inch) "Sugar-Free Shortbread Crumb
    Crust," p. 256
2 cups assorted fresh fruit (sliced
    strawberries, blueberries, sliced
    peaches, sliced bananas)

1. Mix sour cream and sugar substitute. Spread
    on bottom of pie crust. Arrange fresh fruit
    on top. Cut into 8 wedges.

Nutrition Facts	
Serving Size ⅛ pie	
Servings Per Recipe 8	
Amount Per Serving	
Calories 170	
Total Fat 9g	
Cholesterol 19mg	
Sodium 129mg	
Total Carbohydrate 19g	
Dietary Fiber 2g	
Sugars 4g	
Protein 4g	

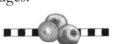

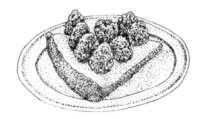

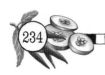
Yummy Lemon Pie

1 (.3 ounce) package instant sugar-free lemon
    gelatin mix
1 teaspoon grated lemon peel plus 1 tablespoon
    lemon juice
1 (8 ounce) carton sugar-free whipped topping,
    thawed
1 (9 inch) "Reduced-Fat Graham Cracker
    Crust," p. 257

Nutrition Facts	
Serving Size ⅛ wedge	
Servings Per Recipe 8	
Amount Per Serving	
Calories 186	
Total Fat 10g	
Cholesterol 15mg	
Sodium 125mg	
Total Carbohydrate 22g	
Dietary Fiber 0g	
Sugars 5g	
Protein 1g	

1. Mix gelatin with ¾ cup boiling water and stir
    continuously until it dissolves. Stir in lemon
    peel and juice and refrigerate until partly set.

2. Stir whipped topping into gelatin and transfer to crust. Refrigerate
    3 to 4 hours.

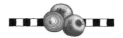

*The easiest way to finely grate citrus peel is
to use a new tool called a microplane, a long fine
grater with a handle.*

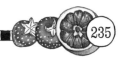

Lime Dream Pie

1 (.3 ounce) box instant sugar-free lime
    gelatin mix
2 cups reduced-fat lime-flavored yogurt
2 cups frozen sugar-free whipped topping,
    thawed
1 (9 inch) "Sugar-Free Chocolate Crumb
    Crust," p. 256

Nutrition Facts
Serving Size ⅛ pie
Servings Per Recipe 8
Amount Per Serving
Calories 172
Total Fat 24g
Cholesterol 17mg
Sodium 147mg
Total Carbohydrate 20g
Dietary Fiber 2g
Sugars 4g
Protein 28g

1. Add gelatin mix to 1 cup boiling water and
   stir to dissolve. Cool to room temperature.

2. Stir yogurt into gelatin and whisk to blend.
   Stir in topping until mixture is smooth.

3. Spoon mixture into crust and refrigerate until set. Cut into
   8 wedges.

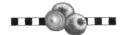

Should I buy sugar-free instead of fat-free frozen whipped topping? Actually, a serving size of 2 tablespoons of fat-free, reduced-fat and sugar-free toppings all contain 3g carbohydrates. Two tablespoons of fat-free and reduced-fat topping have 1g sugars compared to 0g sugars in sugar-free topping. Fat-free is the choice for lower calories — 15 as compared to 20.

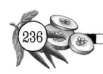

Vanilla Cream Puffs

2 tablespoons butter
½ cup flour
2 eggs
4 (½ cup) sugar-free vanilla pudding
    snack cups

Nutrition Facts	
Serving Size 1 cream puff	
Servings Per Recipe 8	
Amount Per Serving	
Calories 102	
Total Fat 5g	
Cholesterol 61mg	
Sodium 113mg	
Total Carbohydrate 12g	
Dietary Fiber 0g	
Sugars 0g	
Protein 3g	

1. Preheat oven to 400°.

2. In 2-quart saucepan, bring butter and ½ cup water to a boil. Add flour all at once, stir vigorously.

3. Cook and stir over medium heat until mixture forms a ball. Remove from heat. Cool for 10 minutes.

4. Add eggs, one at a time and beat well after each addition. Drop mixture in 8 mounds on sprayed baking sheet.

5. Bake 30 minutes or until golden brown. Transfer to wire rack to cool.

6. Cut tops from puffs and remove soft dough inside. Spoon ¼ cup pudding into cream puff bottoms and replace tops.

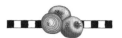

Corn syrup is made when cornstarch is broken down by acids, resulting in a clear, mildly sweet liquid.

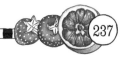
Dark Chocolate-Raspberry Filos

2 (2 ounce) packages frozen mini filo
(phyllo) shells
4 (½ cup) sugar-free dark chocolate pudding
snack cups
1½ cups fresh raspberries

1. Heat filo shells according to package
   directions.

2. Spoon 2 teaspoons pudding into each filo and
   top with 1 or 2 raspberries.

Nutrition Facts
Serving Size 2 shells
Servings Per Recipe 14
Amount Per Serving
Calories 56
Total Fat 3g
Cholesterol 0mg
Sodium 51mg
Total Carbohydrate 9g
Dietary Fiber 1g
Sugars 1g
Protein 1g

*Good news: Dark chocolate with at least
70% cocoa is chock full of antioxidants which are
important for overall health.*

Cherry Pie Filos

1 (2 ounce) package frozen mini filo
(phyllo) shells
1 cup canned reduced-sugar cherry pie filling
Sugar substitute equal to 1 tablespoon sugar
5 tablespoons frozen reduced-fat whipped
topping, thawed

1. Heat filo shells according to package
   directions.

2. Combine pie filling and sugar substitute and
   spoon 1 teaspoon filling into each shell. Top
   with 1 teaspoon whipped topping.

Nutrition Facts
Serving Size 2 shells
Servings Per Recipe 7
Amount Per Serving
Calories 26
Total Fat 1g
Cholesterol 0mg
Sodium 9mg
Total Carbohydrate 5g
Dietary Fiber 0g
Sugars 2g
Protein 0g

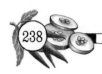
Chocolate Cream Cheese Swirl

4 ounces (½ cup) reduced-fat cream cheese,
   softened
1 (1 ounce) package instant sugar-free fat-free
   chocolate pudding mix
2 cups fat-free milk
¼ cup toasted chopped pecans

Nutrition Facts	
Serving Size ½ cup	
Servings Per Recipe 5	
Amount Per Serving	
Calories 158	
Total Fat 9g	
Cholesterol 18mg	
Sodium 388mg	
Total Carbohydrate 14g	
Dietary Fiber 2g	
Sugars 7g	
Protein 7g	

1. Beat cream cheese until very smooth.

2. Whisk pudding mix and milk in large bowl until it thickens. Stir in cream cheese and gently swirl to mix.

3. Pour into 5 dessert dishes and sprinkle pecans on top.

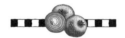

Toasting brings out the true flavor of nuts. To toast in the oven, spread nuts on an ungreased, shallow baking pan. Bake uncovered at 350° for 6 to 10 minutes, stirring frequently, until nuts are light brown and you can smell the toasted aroma.

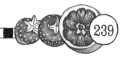
Chocolate Mocha Pudding

1 (1 ounce) package instant sugar-free
   chocolate pudding mix
½ cup strong brewed decaffeinated coffee, cold
1½ cups fat-free milk
4 tablespoons sugar-free frozen whipped
   topping, thawed

Nutrition Facts	
Serving Size ½ cup	
Servings Per Recipe 4	
Amount Per Serving	
Calories 71	
Total Fat 1g	
Cholesterol 0mg	
Sodium 349mg	
Total Carbohydrate 12g	
Dietary Fiber 0g	
Sugars 5g	
Protein 3g	

1. Whisk pudding mix, coffee and milk in
   medium bowl until mixture thickens. Pour ½
   cup pudding into 4 small bowls.

2. Refrigerate about 15 minutes. Spoon
   1 tablespoon whipped topping on top
   before serving.

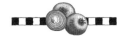

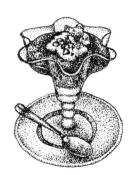

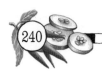

Primo Pistachio Pudding

1 pint sugar-free vanilla ice cream, softened
⅓ cup heavy (whipping) cream
1 (1 ounce) package instant sugar-free pistachio
    pudding mix
1 tablespoon chopped pistachios

1. Slowly beat ice cream, heavy cream, ⅔ cup water and pudding mix in electric mixer or food processor.

2. Spoon into 4 dessert dishes and refrigerate until set. Sprinkle with pistachios.

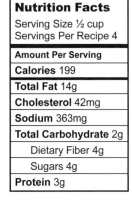

Nutrition Facts
Serving Size ½ cup
Servings Per Recipe 4
Amount Per Serving
Calories 199
Total Fat 14g
Cholesterol 42mg
Sodium 363mg
Total Carbohydrate 2g
Dietary Fiber 4g
Sugars 4g
Protein 3g

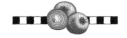

When shopping for milk, nonfat milk may also be called fat-free, skim, zero-fat or no-fat. Low-fat milk refers to 1% milk. Reduced-fat milk refers to 2% milk.

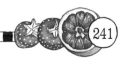

Mandarin-Macadamia Pudding

6 (½ cup) sugar-free vanilla pudding
    snack cups
¼ teaspoon orange or almond extract
1 (11 ounce) can mandarin oranges, drained
2 tablespoons chopped roasted
    macadamia nuts

1. Stir extract into pudding and fold in
   mandarin oranges.

2. Spoon ½ cup pudding into 4 dessert
   dishes and garnish with macadamias.

Nutrition Facts	
Serving Size ½ cup	
Servings Per Recipe 8	
Amount Per Serving	
Calories 96	
Total Fat 3g	
Cholesterol 0mg	
Sodium 144mg	
Total Carbohydrate 15g	
Dietary Fiber less than 1g	
Sugars 6g	
Protein 1g	

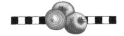

Coconut Pudding

2 cups fat-free milk
1 (1 ounce) package instant sugar-free vanilla
    pudding mix
¼ teaspoon coconut extract
2 tablespoons shredded coconut, toasted

1. In blender, process milk, pudding mix and
   coconut extract.

2. Divide among 4 dessert dishes and sprinkle
   with coconut.

Nutrition Facts	
Serving Size ½ cup	
Servings Per Recipe 4	
Amount Per Serving	
Calories 69	
Total Fat 1g	
Cholesterol 2mg	
Sodium 150mg	
Total Carbohydrate 9g	
Dietary Fiber 0g	
Sugars 7g	
Protein 5g	

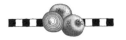

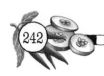

Apricot Cloud

1 (15 ounce) can apricot halves in light syrup,
    rinsed, drained
1 (8 ounce) carton sugar-free frozen whipped
    topping, thawed, divided
¼ teaspoon almond extract

Nutrition Facts	
Serving Size ½ cup	
Servings Per Recipe 6	
Amount Per Serving	
Calories 94	
Total Fat 4g	
Cholesterol 0mg	
Sodium 2mg	
Total Carbohydrate 15g	
Dietary Fiber 0g	
Sugars 3g	
Protein 0g	

1. Add apricots, ½ cup whipped topping and almond extract to food processor. Pulse until apricots are pureed.

2. Fold apricot mixture into remaining whipped topping. Refrigerate 30 minutes. Spoon ½ cup into 6 dessert dishes.

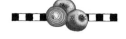

Adding small amounts of nuts and seeds to recipes add crunch and flavor, but they can be high in fat, so don't overdo the sprinkling!

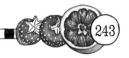
Blueberry Berry

Sugar substitute equal to 3 tablespoons sugar
2 cups fresh blueberries, divided
2 (6 ounce) cartons reduced-fat blueberry
    yogurt
½ teaspoon almond extract

1. Sprinkle sugar substitute on blueberries in medium bowl and toss lightly. Set aside ½ cup blueberries.

2. Mix yogurt and almond extract and toss lightly with 1½ cups blueberries. Spoon ½ cup into 4 dessert dishes and garnish with reserved blueberries.

Nutrition Facts
Serving Size ½ cup
Servings Per Recipe 4
Amount Per Serving
Calories 97
Total Fat 0g
Cholesterol 1mg
Sodium 3mg
Total Carbohydrate 21g
Dietary Fiber 2g
Sugars 14g
Protein 4g

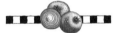

Chocolate Yogo Pops

2 cups fat-free plain yogurt
½ cup "Sugar-Free Hot Cocoa Mix," p. 62
4 (6 ounce) paper cups
4 wooden ice cream sticks

1. Mix yogurt and cocoa mix and spoon into paper cups.

2. Place paper cups in muffin pan and insert stick into each cup. Freeze until hard.

Nutrition Facts
Serving Size ½ cup
Servings Per Recipe 4
Amount Per Serving
Calories 80
Total Fat 0g
Cholesterol 3mg
Sodium 81mg
Total Carbohydrate 14g
Dietary Fiber 0g
Sugars 10g
Protein 5g

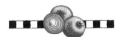

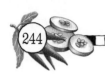

Strawberry-Pistachio Parfait

2 cups fat-free milk
1 (1 ounce) package instant sugar-free pistachio
    pudding mix
2 cups sliced fresh strawberries
4 tablespoons sugar-free chocolate syrup

Nutrition Facts
Serving Size 1 parfait
Servings Per Recipe 4
Amount Per Serving
Calories 124
Total Fat 0g
Cholesterol 2mg
Sodium 161mg
Total Carbohydrate 25g
Dietary Fiber 2g
Sugars 10g
Protein 6g

1. Process milk and pudding mix in blender or
    food processor until mixture thickens. Pour
    into medium bowl and refrigerate until set.

2. Layer ¼ cup pudding and ¼ cup strawberries
    in 4 parfait or stemmed glasses. Repeat
    with layer of ¼ cup pudding and ¼ cup
    strawberries. Drizzle chocolate syrup on top before serving.

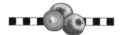

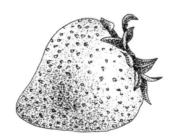

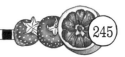

Fais Do-Do Parfait

In Louisiana tradition, a "fais do-do" (fay dough-dough) was a Cajun dance party that went on after the small children were put to bed in a back room. "Fais do-do" is a Cajun French phrase meaning "go to sleep". Today, the term is used in New Orleans to refer to a street dance.

Nutrition Facts	
Serving Size 1¼ cups	
Servings Per Recipe 4	
Amount Per Serving	
Calories 98	
Total Fat 1g	
Cholesterol 3mg	
Sodium 63mg	
Total Carbohydrate 21g	
Dietary Fiber 2g	
Sugars 14g	
Protein 4g	

2 (6 ounce) cartons reduced-fat vanilla yogurt
1-2 teaspoons sugar-free fruit drink powder
2 cups bite-size mixed fresh fruit (berries,
  banana, melon)
4 tablespoons reduced-fat frozen whipped
  topping, thawed

1. Mix yogurt and drink powder in small mixing bowl.

2. Layer ¼ cup yogurt and 2 tablespoons fruit in 4 parfait or stemmed glasses. Repeat with layer of ¼ cup yogurt and 2 tablespoons fruit. Top with 1 tablespoon whipped topping.

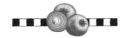

Diabetes professionals have identified a "free food" for diabetics as any food or drink that contains less then 5g carbohydrate and less than 20 calories per serving. However, you are not advised to load up every day on "free foods."

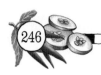

Raspberry Almond Delight

1 (.3 ounce) package instant sugar-free
   raspberry gelatin mix
1 cup sugar-free vanilla ice cream
1 cup raspberries
¼ cup chopped almonds, toasted

Nutrition Facts
Serving Size ½ cup
Servings Per Recipe 6
Amount Per Serving
Calories 130
Total Fat 8g
Cholesterol 15mg
Sodium 115mg
Total Carbohydrate 16g
Dietary Fiber 6g
Sugars 5g
Protein 4g

1. Mix gelatin with 1 cup boiling water and stir until it dissolves completely. Whisk in ice cream.

2. Refrigerate about 20 minutes or until it thickens slightly.

3. Stir in raspberries and almonds. Divide among 6 dessert dishes and refrigerate until firm.

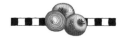

Can people with diabetes eat sweets or chocolate? Yes, if eaten as part of a healthy meal plan and exercise program. Sweets are no more "off limits" to people with diabetes than they are to people without diabetes.

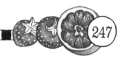
Caramel Apples

2 medium tart apples
4 tablespoons sugar-free caramel syrup
4 tablespoons reduced-fat frozen whipped
    topping, thawed

Nutrition Facts	
Serving Size ½ apple Servings Per Recipe 4	
Amount Per Serving	
Calories 94	
Total Fat 1g	
Cholesterol 0mg	
Sodium 33mg	
Total Carbohydrate 24g	
Dietary Fiber 1g	
Sugars 9g	
Protein 0g	

1. Preheat oven to 350°.

2. Peel and halve apples. Use a melon baller to remove apple cores. Spray baking dish and place apples and ⅓ cup water in dish.

3. Bake, uncovered, for 40 minutes or until apples become tender. Remove from oven and place apple halves on 4 dessert plates.

4. Drizzle 1 tablespoon syrup onto each apple half and top with whipped topping.

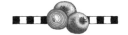

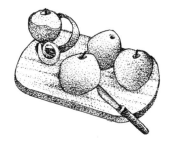

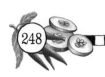

Love-It Cinnamon Apples

2 medium apples, peeled, coarsely chopped
1 tablespoon packed brown sugar
½ teaspoon ground cinnamon
2 teaspoons lemon juice

Nutrition Facts	
Serving Size ½ cup Servings Per Recipe 4	
Amount Per Serving	
Calories 53	
Total Fat 0g	
Cholesterol 0mg	
Sodium 1mg	
Total Carbohydrate 14g	
Dietary Fiber 1g	
Sugars 12g	
Protein 0g	

1. Pour ½ cup water, apples, brown sugar and cinnamon in 2 to 3-quart saucepan. Bring to a boil and reduce heat to low.

2. Simmer, covered, about 20 minutes or until apples are soft.

3. Remove apples from pan and bring liquid to a boil. Reduce heat to medium and cook until liquid thickens.

4. Stir in lemon juice and apples and heat through.

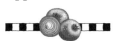

If your brown sugar has hardened, seal it in a plastic bag with a wedge of apple for 1 to 2 days.

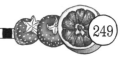

Spicy Baked Apples

2 medium tart apples, halved, cored
Granular sugar-substitute equal to
    4 teaspoons sugar
½ teaspoon apple pie spice
¼ cup frozen whipped topping, thawed,
    divided

Nutrition Facts		
Serving Size ½ apple		
Servings Per Recipe 4		
Amount Per Serving		
Calories 58		
Total Fat 1g		
Cholesterol 0mg		
Sodium 1mg		
Total Carbohydrate 14g		
Dietary Fiber 2g		
Sugars 9g		
Protein 0g		

1. Preheat oven to 350°.

2. Arrange apple halves, cut side up, in
   9 x 9-inch baking dish. Add ½ cup water.

3. Combine sugar-substitute and apple pie
   spice and spoon into center of apple halves.

4. Cover with foil and bake about 45 minutes or until apples are
   tender. Remove apples and transfer liquid in baking dish to
   small saucepan.

5. Bring to a boil, reduce heat, and simmer until most of liquid
   evaporates.

6. Pour over baked apple halves and spoon 1 tablespoon whipped
   topping on top of each apple half.

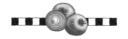

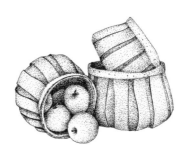

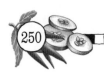

Peach-Ricotta Dessert

2 cups sliced fresh peaches or frozen
    unsweetened sliced peaches, thawed,
    drained
1 cup fat-free ricotta cheese
½ teaspoon almond or vanilla extract
Sugar substitute equal to 2 tablespoons sugar

1. Divide peaches among 6 dessert bowls.
Combine ricotta, extract and sugar substitute
in bowl and spoon over peaches.

Nutrition Facts	
Serving Size ½ cup	
Servings per recipe 6	
Amount Per Serving	
Calories 90	
Total Fat 0g	
Cholesterol 0mg	
Sodium 60mg	
Total Carbohydrate 12g	
Dietary Fiber 1g	
Sugars 10g	
Protein 11g	

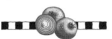

Snack: Dip banana slices in orange juice and freeze on a baking sheet until hard. Store in a freezer-proof plastic bag.

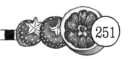
Peaches and Cream

2 cups fresh or unsweetened frozen peaches,
    thawed, cut in chunks
Sugar substitute equal to 2 teaspoons sugar
2 (6 ounce) cartons reduced-fat peach yogurt
6 tablespoons reduced-fat frozen whipped
    topping, thawed

1. Sprinkle peaches with sugar substitute. Fold
   yogurt and whipped topping together.

2. Layer ¼ cup yogurt mixture and
   2 tablespoons peaches in 5 dessert bowls.
   Repeat with layer of ¼ cup yogurt mixture
   and 2 tablespoons peaches.

Nutrition Facts
Serving Size 1 cup
Servings Per Recipe 5
Amount Per Serving
Calories 76
Total Fat 1g
Cholesterol 1mg
Sodium 46mg
Total Carbohydrate 15g
Dietary Fiber 1g
Sugars 10g
Protein 3g

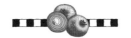

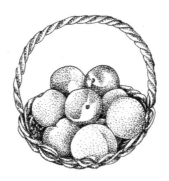

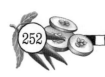

Fresh Fruit Cup

2 cups chopped apple with peel
1 cup sliced red grapes
1 kiwi, quartered, sliced
1 banana, peeled, sliced

1. Mix all ingredients in large bowl and spoon ½ cup into 7 dessert dishes.

Nutrition Facts
Serving Size ½ cup
Servings Per Recipe 7
Amount Per Serving
Calories 56
Total Fat 0g
Cholesterol 0mg
Sodium 1mg
Total Carbohydrate 14g
Dietary Fiber 2g
Sugars 10g
Protein 1g

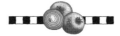

Family Fruit Delight

2 (15 ounce) cans no-sugar-added sliced
   peaches in water, drained
1 (20 ounce) can pineapple tidbits in juice,
   drained
1 (11 ounce) can mandarin oranges in light
   syrup, drained
2 (6 ounce) cartons fat-free reduced-sugar
   peach yogurt

1. Cut peaches into chunks. Mix peach chunks with remaining ingredients in large bowl and gently stir together.

Nutrition Facts
Serving size ½ cup
Servings Per Recipe 12
Amount Per Serving
Calories 66
Total Fat 0g
Cholesterol 1mg
Sodium 19mg
Total Carbohydrate 15g
Dietary Fiber 1g
Sugars 14g
Protein 1g

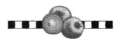

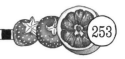

Citrus-Honey Melon Cups

2 medium limes
2 tablespoons honey
4 cups (1 inch) cubed melon*

1. Grate 1 tablespoon lime peel and squeeze 2 to 3 teaspoons fresh lime juice. Combine juice with honey.

2. Divide melon among 4 dessert bowls. Drizzle with lime honey mixture and garnish with lime peel.

TIP: Watermelon, honeydew or cantaloupe are all great in this recipe.

Nutrition Facts	
Serving Size 1 cup	
Servings Per Recipe 4	
Amount Per Serving	
Calories 92	
Total Fat 0g	
Cholesterol 0mg	
Sodium 26mg	
Total Carbohydrate 19g	
Dietary Fiber 2g	
Sugars 17g	
Protein 1g	

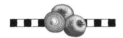

The flavor of cantaloupe and honeydew melons is greatly enhanced by sprinkling with lime juice.

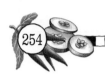

Purple Plum Dessert Sauce

Serve this dessert sauce over sugar-free angel food cake or sugar-free ice cream for a delicious treat!

1 tablespoon cornstarch
Sugar substitute equal to ½ cup sugar
1 pound purple plums, pits removed, sliced
1 tablespoon lemon juice

Nutrition Facts	
Serving Size ¼ cup	
Servings Per Recipe 12	
Amount Per Recipe	
Calories 20	
Total Fat 0g	
Cholesterol 0mg	
Sodium 3mg	
Total Carbohydrate 5g	
Dietary Fiber 1g	
Sugars 4g	
Protein 0g	

1. Mix cornstarch and sugar substitute in 2 to 3-quart saucepan. Stir in plums and lemon juice.

2. Bring to a boil, reduce heat and simmer 8 to 10 minutes.

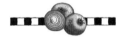

Locate sugar-free breakfast and dessert syrups at the grocery store. The carbohydrate content is lower than regular sugar. Check the calories — if it's 20 calories or less per serving, it's a good choice for you.

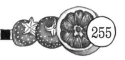
Berry Dessert Sauce

2 cups fresh berries*
1 tablespoon packed brown sugar
2 teaspoons cornstarch
1 tablespoon lemon juice

Nutrition Facts		
Serving Size 3 tablespoons Servings Per Recipe 8		
Amount Per Serving		
Calories 35		
Total Fat 0g		
Cholesterol 0mg		
Sodium 1mg		
Total Carbohydrate 9g		
Dietary Fiber 1g		
Sugars 6g		
Protein 0g		

1. Wash berries just before use. Use small berries whole. Hull and slice strawberries.

2. Dissolve brown sugar in ½ cup water in 2 to 3-quart saucepan. Add berries and bring to a boil. Quickly reduce heat and simmer until berries are soft, about 5 minutes.

3. Remove ¼ cup hot juice and cool slightly. Stir in cornstarch until it dissolves and transfer back to saucepan.

4. Bring to a simmer and stir until mixture thickens, about 1 minute. Stir in lemon juice.

TIP: *Use any of your favorite berries or those growing in your backyard. You'll love this recipe.*

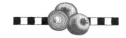

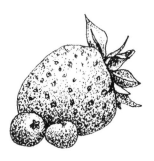

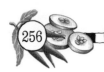

Sugar-Free Shortbread Crumb Crust

1¼ cups sugar-free shortbread cookie crumbs
¼ cup melted butter

1. Preheat oven to 325°.

2. Mix crumbs and melted butter. Press firmly in 9-inch pie plate.

3. Bake for about 6 minutes. Cool completely before using.

Nutrition Facts	
Serving Size ⅛ crust	
Servings Per Recipe 8	
Amount Per Serving	
Calories 132	
Total Fat 9g	
Cholesterol 15mg	
Sodium 88mg	
Total Carbohydrate 13g	
Dietary Fiber 1g	
Sugars 0g	
Protein 1g	

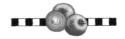

Sugar-Free Chocolate Crumb Crust

1¼ cups sugar-free chocolate cookie crumbs
¼ cup melted butter

1. Preheat oven to 325°.

2. Mix crumbs and melted butter. Press firmly in 9-inch pie plate.

3. Bake for about 6 minutes. Cool completely before using.

Nutrition Facts	
Serving Size ⅛ crust	
Servings Per Recipe 8	
Amount Per Serving	
Calories 101	
Total Fat 21g	
Cholesterol 15mg	
Sodium 79mg	
Total Carbohydrate 10g	
Dietary Fiber 2g	
Sugars 0g	
Protein 1g	

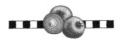

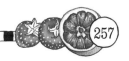

Reduced-Fat Graham Cracker Crust

1¼ cups reduced-fat graham cracker crumbs
¼ cup melted butter

1. Preheat oven to 325°.

2. Mix crumbs and melted butter. Press firmly in 9-inch pie plate. Bake for about 6 minutes. Cool completely before using.

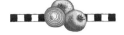

Nutrition Facts		
Serving Size ⅛ crust		
Servings Per Recipe 8		
Amount Per Serving		
Calories 130		
Total Fat 7g		
Cholesterol 15		
Sodium 125mg		
Total Carbohydrate 16g		
Dietary Fiber 1g		
Sugars 5g		
Protein 1g		

We hope everyone recognizes the importance of sharing time and meals together. If you do, our families will be stronger, our nation will be stronger and our own little part of the world will feel a little safer and a little more loving.

The Publisher

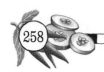

Index

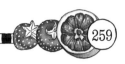

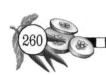

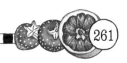

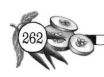
Chicken

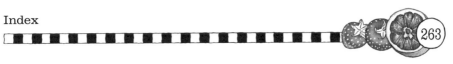
Chilies – See Peppers

Chocolate

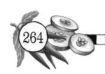

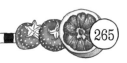

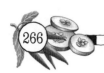

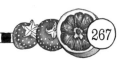

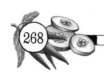

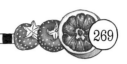

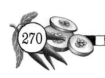

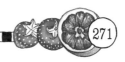

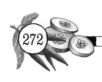

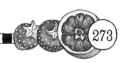

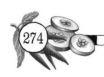

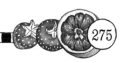

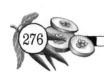

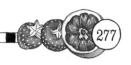

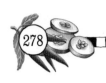

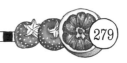

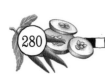

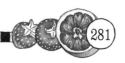

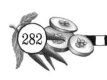
Cookbooks Published by Cookbook Resources, LLC
Bringing Family and Friends to the Table

The Best 1001 Short, Easy Recipes
1001 Slow Cooker Recipes
1001 Short, Easy, Inexpensive Recipes
1001 Fast Easy Recipes
1001 America's Favorite Recipes
1001 Easy Inexpensive Grilling Recipes
1,001 Easy Potluck Recipes
Easy Slow Cooker Cookbook
Busy Woman's Slow Cooker Recipes
Busy Woman's Quick & Easy Recipes
365 Easy Soups and Stews
365 Easy Chicken Recipes
365 Easy One-Dish Recipes
365 Easy Soup Recipes
365 Easy Vegetarian Recipes
365 Easy Casserole Recipes
365 Easy Pasta Recipes
365 Easy Slow Cooker Recipes
Super Simple Cupcake Recipes
Leaving Home Cookbook and Survival Guide
Essential 3-4-5 Ingredient Recipes
Ultimate 4 Ingredient Cookbook
Easy Cooking with 5 Ingredients
The Best of Cooking with 3 Ingredients
Easy Diabetic Recipes
Ultimate 4 Ingredient Diabetic Cookbook
4-Ingredient Recipes for 30-Minute Meals
Cooking with Beer
The Washington Cookbook
The Pennsylvania Cookbook
The California Cookbook
Best-Loved Canadian Recipes
Best-Loved Recipes from the Pacific Northwest
Easy Homemade Preserves (Handbook with Photos)
Garden Fresh Recipes (Handbook with Photos)

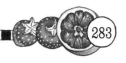

cookbook
resources LLC
www.cookbookresources.com
Toll-Free 866-229-2665
Your Ultimate Source for Easy Cookbooks

Cookbooks for Cooking and Reading Entertainment

Cookbooks Are Handbooks...

65+ easy recipes with 65+ color photographs are packed into each convenient, easy-to-carry handbook. Simple, practical recipes with everyday ingredients and fun highlights are perfect for busy cooks and everyone who likes to read cookbooks. Designed to be easy to use and read, these full-color books open flat on your countertop without taking up lots of space.

Size 5 x 7¼   176 pages
Color Photos   Hard Cover
Concealed Wire Binding

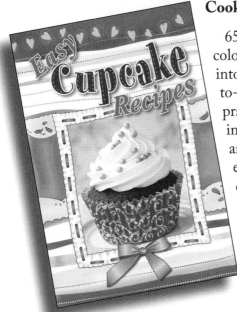

Easy Cupcake Recipes – It's fun for the whole family! Short prep times, quick baking times without fancy ingredients and lots of ideas for basic, inexpensive decorating make this book great rain-or-shine entertainment!

Cool Smoothies – These recipes are fast... fun... and good for you. Great on-the-go meals and snacks are the best substitute for milkshakes and "fat snacks". These recipes have fewer calories, more vitamins and minerals, and delicious low-fat options. Perfect for icy beverages and for picky eaters!

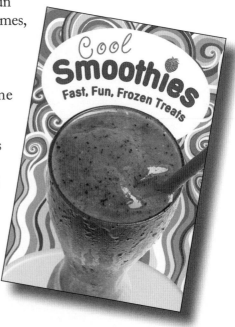

Cookbooks for Cooking and Reading Entertainment

Designed to be easy to use and read, these full-color books open flat on your countertop without taking up lots of space.

Size 5 x 7¼   176 pages
Color Photos   Hard Cover
Concealed Wire Binding

Easy Homemade Preserves – Make the most of your food dollar by preserving fresh fruits and vegetables from your own family garden or from local farmers… and make them

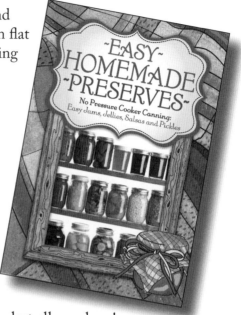

last all year long! No pressure cooker needed… use simple hot water bath method.

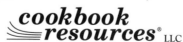

Garden Fresh Recipes – Buying food from locally grown sources is the best way to give your family the highest quality fruits and vegetables. Fresh from your own garden or from your local farmers' market, fruits and vegetables are at their tastiest and healthiest. These easy and delicious recipes make family meals memorable.!

1001 Recipes Collections!

Each cookbook features 1001 of our best, easiest and most practical recipes using everyday ingredients. These cookbooks are great for beginners and advanced cooks alike. Recipes are easy to read and easy to follow, and content is fun and entertaining. You go home with a bargain when you buy 1001 great-tasting recipes.

Paperback   Size 6 x 9
Hard Cover   Comb Binding
Size 6½ x 9¼

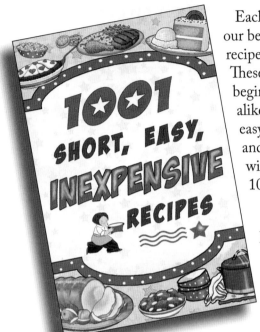

1001 Short, Easy, Inexpensive Recipes not only gives recipes and tips to save money, it also helps us with meals for busy families with many recipes with just 3 to 5 ingredients. This cookbook gives you great choices for making family meal memorable. (400 pages)

1001 Fast Easy Recipes is your quick-look cookbook for easy-to-prepare meals made with ingredients right from your own pantry! Spend less time cooking and more time with friends and family enjoying the meals you have created. (400 pages)

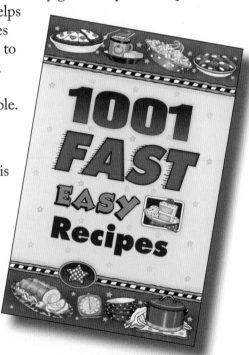

1001 Recipes Collections!

1001 Slow Cooker Recipes – Life just got easier! Put your food inside a slow cooker, cover the pot, turn the switch to "on" Come home after hours of errands, soccer games, meetings, work or play and dinner is ready! Meals are simple, convenient and much better than fast food! These recipes are so easy anyone can cook them and they are so delicious everyone will love them. (416 pages)

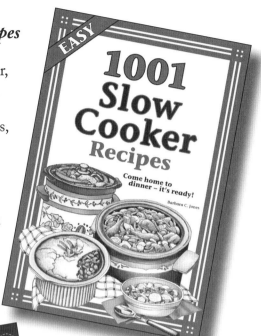

Essential 3-4-5 Ingredient Cookbook is three cookbooks in one! Featuring the best of great recipes with 3 ingredients, 4 ingredients and 5 ingredients, these cookbooks offer ways to create quick and terrific meals. Using ingredients from your pantry, this cookbook is as simple as it gets! (480 pages)

cookbook resources ® LLC
www.cookbookresources.com
Toll-free 1-866-229-2665
Your Ultimate Source for Easy Cookbooks

Eating Right Is Fun and Easy!

Filled with recipes that are easy, delicious and good for you, each of these cookbooks includes nutritional information with every recipe to let you know exactly what you're eating! (Each has 288 pages.)

Hard Cover   Semi-concealed Wire Binding
      Size 7¼ x 9¼
Paperback   Size 6 x 9
Hard Cover   Comb Bound   Size 6½ x 9¼

Ultimate 4 Ingredient Diabetic Cookbook – You don't have to sacrifice flavor or convenience when you cook these healthy, delicious recipes that your family will love. It's easy when you use only 4 ingredients!

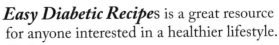

Easy Diabetic Recipes is a great resource for anyone interested in a healthier lifestyle. Delicious, easy-to-prepare dishes that everyone likes make good eating habits easy for your entire family.

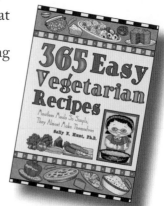

Enjoy good food that's good for you and your family with *365 Easy Vegetarian Recipes.* Featuring delicious, healthy, short and simple recipes, it includes up-to-date revised favorites from appetizers to desserts.

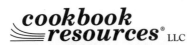

cookbook
≋resources ® LLC
www.cookbookresources.com
Toll-free 1-866-229-2665
Your Ultimate Source for Easy Cookbooks